HERBS &
AROMATHERAPY

FOR THE

Reproductive System

MEN AND WOMEN

Jeanne Rose

Frog, Ltd.
Berkeley, California

Herbs & Aromatherapy for the Reproductive System
Copyright © 1994 by Jeanne Rose. No portion of this book, except for brief review, may be reproduced in any form without written permission of the publisher. For information contact Frog, Ltd. c/o North Atlantic Books.

Published by Frog, Ltd.

Frog, Ltd. books are distributed by
North Atlantic Books
P.O. Box 12327
Berkeley, California 94712

Cover and book design by Paula Morrison
Typeset by Catherine Campaigne

Printed in the United States of America

Library of Congress Cataloging-in-Publication Data

Rose, Jeanne, 1940–
    Herbs for the reproductive system / Jeanne Rose.
        p.   cm.
    Includes bibliographical references.
    ISBN 1–883319–17–X
    1. Generative organs—Diseases—Alternative treatment.
    2. Herbs—Therapeutic use.   I. Title
    RC877.R73   1994
    616.6'506—dc20   94-19980
                                                                CIP

2   3   4   5   6   7   8   9   /   98   97   96   95

HERBS &
AROMATHERAPY
FOR THE
Reproductive System

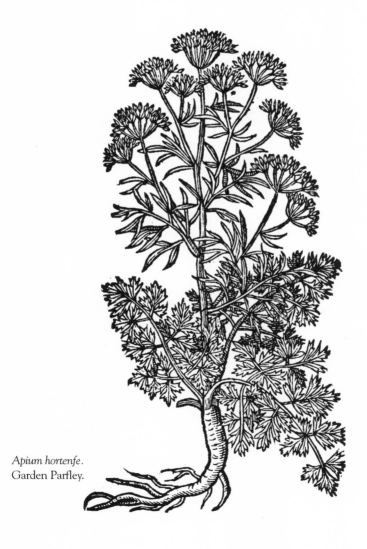

Apium hortenfe.
Garden Parfley.

Publisher's Caution

All plants and their essential oils, like all medicines, may be harmful and even dangerous if used improperly—if they are taken internally when prescribed for external use, if they are taken in excess, or if they are taken for too long a time. Allergic reactions and unpredictable sensitivities or illness may develop. There are other factors to consider as well: since the strength of wild herbs and various essential oils varies, knowledge of their growing conditions and distillation methods is helpful. Be sure your herbs are fresh and whole and your essential oils are not contaminated with foreign objects like melting rubber stoppers. Keep conditions of use as sterile as possible.

We do not advocate, endorse, or guarantee the curative effects of any of the substances listed in this book. We have made every effort to see that any botanical that is dangerous or potentially dangerous has been noted as such. When you use plants and their essential oils, recognize their potency and use them with care. Medical consultation is recommended for those recipes marked as dangerous.

The botanical names listed under each herb and essential oil do not always refer to one species only, but may also apply to others, which in herbal medicine have been recognized as substitutes.

Here, as in all her herbals, Jeanne Rose follows ancient tradition and capitalizes the names of the plants that are used therapeutically in herbalism, including such items as Coffee and Apricots. This is to make them stand out, give them substance, and to show that all herbs, and foods as well, can be used as therapy.

Acknowledgments

For suggestions about the shape and content of this book I owe much to Penelope deVries who also encouraged me to do this series of small books based on Part II of **The Herbal Studies Course** which I call **The Medicinal Herbal**.

I also owe much to all those herbalists and women who have come and gone before me and to the books I frequently refer to from my library.

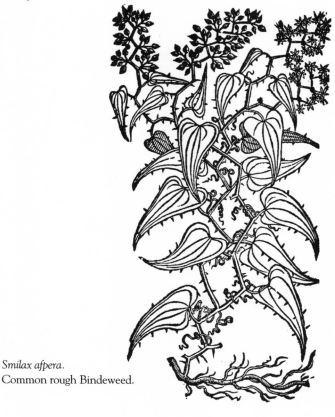

Smilax afpera.
Common rough Bindeweed.

Woman Secret

Silphium, Queen Anne's Lace and Rue
A potion known only by few
For those who are wise
They no longer need compromise
Herbs, knowledge or family size.

May 1994 ...... jeanne colon

Table of Contents

Author's Preface xi

Foreword xii

Part I: The Female

1. Female Basics 3

2. The Menstrual Cycle: The Hormone Cycle. 7
   Natural Birth Control, A Chart of Changes

3. Natural Birth Control: A Summary of Changes 11

4. Twelve Ways Not to Get Pregnant 13
   *The Cervical Cap; The Condom; The Diaphragm;
   Spermicide; The Sponge; Depo-Provera; The Pill;
   The Mini Pill; The IUD; Implants; Female Sterilization;
   Future Contraceptives*

5. Herbs for Females 19

6. Herbal Formulas for Women from Menarch to
   Menopause 23
   *Menstrual Tardiness; Menarch; Aromatherapy for the
   Menarch; Menstrual Regulation; Premenstrual Tension,
   Acne, and Water Retention; Vaginal Infections; Basic
   YEGG Formula, Bolus, and Douche; Aromatherapy
   Treatments for Uterine and Vaginal Infections; Bladder and
   Kidney Infections; A Dietary Plan and Supplements*

7. Colortherapy (The use of color to treat conditions) . . 45
   *The Special Get-Rid-Of-Your-Problem-Within-One-Week
   Therapy*

8. Pregnancy and Childbirth 49
   Aromatherapy Treatments for Pregnancy and Childbirth

9. Seven Steps to Healing Cysts, Vague Aches,
   Menorrhagia 53

10. Menopause 57
    Hot Flashes; Balance the Hormonal Output; Dry Vagina;
    Relieving Emotional States Using Aromatherapy; Aching
    Feet; Women's Health vs. Horses; Simple Formulas During
    Menopause

Notes to Text 67

Part II: The Male

11. Male Basics 73

12. Birth Control 75
    How Not to Get Women Pregnant

13. Herbs for Males 77

14. Herbal Formulas for Men 81
    Cryptorchism; Epididymitis; Lack of Erection or Impotence;
    Orchitis; Prostate Health and Troubles; Scrotal Eczema;
    Spermatorrhea; Venereal Diseases; Venereal Warts and
    Herpes; Herbal Aphrodisiacs

Part III: Helpful Information

Glossary of Herbs 91

Herbs for the Reproductive System 93

Acid-Alkaline Diet and Chart 105

Simple Methods of Preparation 109

Glossary of Terms 115

Source List 121

Bibliography 125

Author's Preface

The subjects of the human reproductive system, the herbs and essential oils that can be used to treat these organs, and the conditions that arise from dysfunction are rich and complex. Rich in folk remedies, herbal remedies, and allopathic remedies, and complex because human beings themselves are complex — cognizant beings whose emotional status often manifests as physiological problems.

This little book is not meant to provide information on every single issue that arises for the organs of reproduction. It touches on fertility problems only briefly and doesn't tackle the issue of AIDS. This book is for the everyday events that arise, discussing such subjects as determining where in the woman's cycle she is fertile, easy-to-use remedies for prostatitis, contraception methods that can be employed by both men and women, fungus and bacterial infections, and the herbal therapy/aromatherapy remedies to use.

You will find Herbal Formulas and Aromatherapy formulas for women from menarche to menopause, for men from aphrodisiacs and aromatherapy to warts and herpes. Vague uterine aches, PMS, and bladder and kidney infections are all mentioned for women, and epididymitis, erection problems, and venereal disease are mentioned for men. The remedies are easily available and easily used; the herbs and essential oils may be obtained by mail order from the Source List in Part III. A glossary of herbs and terms is presented as well.

This book will be a helpful tool in your quest for healthful solutions to everyday problems.

Jeanne Rose
Spring 1994

Foreword

Most books about Female and Male Sexuality and Reproduction have been written by men who don't represent the female reproductive structure with accuracy or intimacy.

Herbs & Aromatherapy for the Reproductive System has been written with emphasis on accuracy and intimacy, particularly when representing the female structure. It has been our goal to demystify genitalia and organic sexual function and to provide gentle care for these fragile parts with the use of herbs and common-sense treatment. Our sex parts have always been treated in a distant, disdainful manner, fostering misunderstanding and malfunction as a result. We believe no matter what you do with your sex parts, they are indeed an integral part of your health and well-being and require at least as much respect as your stomach or skin!

Penelope deVries
Spring 1994

THE FEMALE

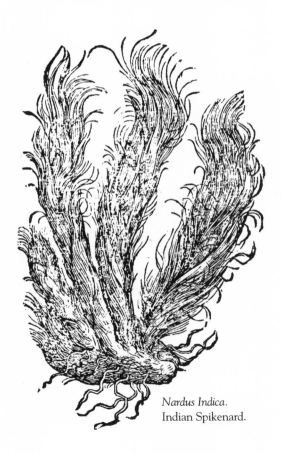

Nardus Indica.
Indian Spikenard.

Notes

Chapter 1

Female Basics

Basic anatomy is—or should be—well-known by all men and women. The sexual organs include the breasts, vagina, and clitoris.

The clitoris is analogous to the tip of the penis; it engorges with blood and enlarges during sexual excitement. An orgasm occurs with proper stimulation. The clitoris is located within the inner lips or inner labia *(labia minora)* at the upper entrance of the outer sexual organs or *labia majora,* near the pubic mound and forward of the vaginal entrance. The urethra, the opening to the bladder, is between the vaginal orifice and the clitoris. Because the clitoral body extends around both sides of the vaginal orifice, one can call this opening the clitoral opening to the vagina. The various parts of the clitoris actually surround and extend along the vagina and are part of its very structure.

The clitoris is a more complicated structure than most anatomy books usually care to describe. The clitoris surrounds and extends along the vagina, varying greatly in size, texture, and color from one woman to the next. It is an area of intense concentration of nerves and blood vessels. This fresh view of female anatomy is detailed in *A New View of a Woman's Body,* by the Federation of Feminist Women's Health Centers (New York: Simon and Schuster, 1981, 1989).

These three structures—clitoris, urethral opening, and clitoral opening to the vagina—are all located within the inner lips, which are surrounded by the outer lips *(labia majora)*.

The reproductive organs include the breasts, vagina, uterus, Fallopian tubes, and ovaries. The vaginal opening or clitoral opening to the vagina leads into the vagina, that muscular tube which encloses the penis during intercourse and is the tunnel through which the baby reaches the outside world.

The walls of the vagina continually change during the changing hormonal menstrual cycle, becoming thicker, somewhat textured, and lighter in color during the estrogen phase or first half of the cycle, and smoother, darker, and rather puffy just prior to menstruation. These changes are highly individual. A woman should carefully examine herself using a speculum throughout her cycle for several cycles to determine exactly what her personal changes are. Look for color changes in the vaginal walls and observe the change in texture from puffy to firm, the smoothness, or the horizontal or vertical ridges.

The vagina "sweats" during sexual arousal, aiding masturbation or actual intercourse. During ovulation this secretion is sugary, more alkaline, and can taste very sweet, inciting oral sex, while during the latter half of the cycle—that is, the progesterone phase—it is less sweet and often has a slightly bitter acid taste.

All of these changes in the vagina, the vulva, the mucous secretions, and the changes that will be mentioned concerning the uterus, the cervix and os (its opening) are indicative of where a woman is in her menstrual cycle. With this information and the rise and fall of her temperature, knowledgeable and observant men and women can determine nearly exactly the time of ovulation and therefore practice natural birth control.

At the upper end of the vagina is the os, the opening of the cervix which opens into the uterus. Upon self-examination, one can feel the cervix as a rather firm, roundish knob with a slit-like opening in the center. It is this opening that is called the os. If it is a slit, it may be in an upturned (smiling) or down-turned (frowning) position. In the course of menstruation, the cervix hangs low in the vaginal canal, the os is somewhat open, and blood oozes out of it. During the next few days in the cycle after the flow and before ovulation, the os is closed and the cervix looks lighter. After ovulation, it becomes darker, even bluish in color.

The cervical mucus ranges from clear to brownish to green-ish to milky to yellow. These variations depend on cyclical changes and whether or not it is a healthy discharge. The consistency is either thick or thin, and stringy, stretchy, or foamy. There can be a lot of mucus or very little. The mucus varies if the birth control pill is used, and certainly if the female is fertile or not. The mucus can have a very mild aroma or an acid one, somewhat like stale yeast. It can be fishy or even sour. During ovulation it smells very mild and rather pleasant; during the last half of the cycle, it can smell rather bitter, sour, or fishy, no doubt due to the progesterone build-up. Before ovulation the mucus is thick, then it clears and thins and becomes stretchy and stringy at ovulation. When it is no longer fertile, the mucus again thickens and gets milky and scant. It has been described at this time as resembling dry, thick paste.

Women and their partners may also notice another phenomenon that indicates ovulation. During the early part of the cycle the cervix can easily be felt hanging down quite low in the vaginal canal, but as ovulation time approaches the cervix moves up, thereby lengthening the vaginal canal. The uterus may be ballooning up and out, pulling the cervix along with it. At this time it is very difficult to feel with the fingers, and deeper penetration can be achieved during intercourse. If the cervical cap is used for birth control, it is much easier for the man, with his longer fingers, to put the cap into place. This also allows him to share in the responsibility of birth control. Intercourse at this time can be vigorous and exciting because of the sweet-

smelling and -tasting secretions and longer "tunnel of love."
After ovulation, during the fourteen days before menstruation,
the cervix again moves down into the vaginal canal and can be
easily felt.

The uterus is considered strictly a reproductive organ. It is
pear-shaped and hollow, with the two Fallopian tubes leading
away from the top. The other end is called the cervix, the thick
muscular structure that opens into the vagina. The uterus is constantly relaxing and contracting slightly. The contractions which
are strong and spasmodic increase during orgasm from the greatly
increased blood supply to the area, causing the uterus to bal-
loon upward which enlarges the vagina, serving to "suck in" the
sperm.

Prior to ovulation the uterine walls increase in size, and
glands lining the wall secrete glucose and other nourishment
for the egg if it is fertilized and implants. After ovulation, if no
fertilization has occurred, the lining of the uterus begins to dis-
integrate. Increased contractions will expel this lining, and this
is the process called the menstrual flow.

At the end of the Fallopian tubes are the ovaries. These two
organs are not connected to the Fallopian tubes but are encir-
cled by the finger-like projections of the tubes. The ovaries have
two functions. They produce ova, or eggs, and they secrete the
two main hormones that define a woman's cycle, estrogen and
progesterone. At birth, a woman's entire complement of ova is
already in place. The ovaries are rather small until puberty, when
they enlarge and ovulation begins.

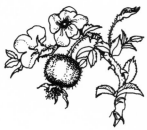

Chapter 2

The Menstrual Cycle: The Hormone Cycle

The menarche is the first menstruation, that time when physical changes occur. The breasts enlarge, the hips round out, the ovaries enlarge and mature, and ovulation occurs. Hormones are released that will subsequently govern the rhythm of a woman's life.

The pituitary secretes follicular stimulating hormone (FSH), which stimulates the Graafian follicles of the ovaries to mature, of which only one will reach full maturity each cycle. When a follicle is nearly mature the Fallopian tube actually moves toward it and picks up the egg as it is pushed out the follicle. In mid-cycle, there is a surge of luteinizing hormone secreted by the pituitary (LH), softening the plug of non-fertile mucus that blocks the cervical opening, triggering ovulation, and stimulating the growth of the *corpus luteum*,* which is the burst follicle which has produced and secreted the egg. As the follicle ruptures, the egg oozes out, and this ovulation can be felt by some women as pain called *Mittleschmertz*. The follicle cells produce estrogen which builds up the *endometrium* (lining) of the uterus.

---

*A small yellow area in an ovary found at the site where an egg has formed and burst from the gland.[1]

7

Natural Birth Control

A Summary of the Changes that Occur in the Body whose Observance Can be Used to Determine When Ovulation has Occurred and Therefore When a Diaphragm, Cervical Cap, or Abstention Should Be Used.

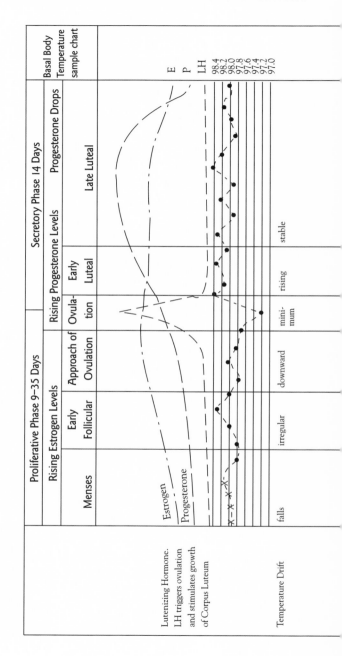

Onset	abrupt	distinct	indistinct	distinct	abrupt	gradual
Length of time	4 days	5 days	4–5 days	1–2 days	3 days	10 days
Variation	3–6 days	1–35 days	4–8 days	slight	4–5 days	9–11 days (ovulation occurs 14 days prior to next menses)
Cervix texture	firm	firm	softening	soft & spongy	firming	firm, almost hard
Position	hanging low	low	moving up	drawn up (out of reach)	lower	lower
Os Large	closed	barely open	more open	gaping	closing	tight
Os Small	closed	closed	dimpling	gaping	closing	closed
Cervical Mucus Appears in Os	blood	opaque plug	thick cordlike	watery	opaque	very dry
Amount	wanes	scanty	increasing	voluminous	decrease	scanty
Clarity	bloody	opaque	streaked	glassy	cloudy	opaque, yellow
Consistency	—	tacky, gummy	ropy	runny, stretchy	tacky	like paste
Scent	—	mild	bland	pleasant	stronger	sour, yeasty or fishy
Taste	—	—	not unpleasant	sweet	less sweet	rather acid, sour
Breasts	—	—	—	sensitive	—	may be sore just prior to menses
Vagina	—	—	walls thicker, textured	—	—	walls—smoother and rather puffy
Color	—	—	may become lighter	—	may get darker	may get darker
Secretions	—	—	become sweeter	sweet	may taste bitter	may taste bitter
Vulva	—	—	may become lighter	—	may get darker	may get darker until the menses
Sexual Desire	stronger	increasingly stronger	increasingly stronger	intense	weaker	may disappear altogether
"Is it Safe?"	yes	yes	decreasingly	no	increasingly yes	increasingly yes

At ovulation the *cilia* (fingerlike projections) in the cervical cysts actually line up vertically to create a "highway" for the sperm. And at ovulation the mucus is more alkaline than at other times, which creates a favorable habitat for sperm. Sperm can live up to five days in this fertile mucus.

The follicle is now called the *corpus luteum* and it produces progesterone for up to eight days. Progesterone stimulates the growth and thickening of the uterine walls in preparation for the implanting of a fertilized egg. The mucus lining thickens and the blood supply to the area is increased. The uterine muscle expands and contracts less because progesterone also inhibits a hormone called *oxytocin*, which stimulates contractions associated with labor. If the egg is not fertilized, the *corpus luteum* degenerates through the influence of another hormone. Progesterone production ceases and the uterine lining is shed. This is called menstruation.

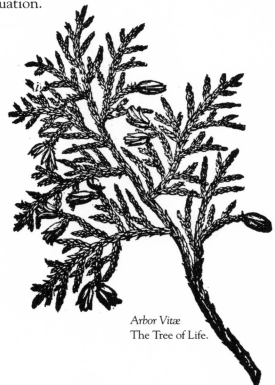

Arbor Vitæ
The Tree of Life.

Chapter 3

Natural Birth Control:
A Summary of Changes

Birth control has unfortunately been of primary concern to women only. Few men have ever taken the time to learn about the changes that occur in a woman that would allow them to know when she ovulates. But men as well as women can examine the vulva, the vagina, and the cervical mucus, and they can taste, touch, and smell these organs and take note of the sensory variations in the secretions to tell where the woman is in her cycle. This is the essential knowledge for natural birth control. No one can tell you exactly what these changes will be, for each woman is unique, her cycle is hers alone.

From menarche to menopause, it is beneficial for an intelligent woman to keep an exact record of her menstrual cycle and the changes in her body. Keep a log or a calendar of your observations. Examine yourself carefully and learn how to use a speculum. With this knowledge pregnancy will never come as a surprise. It will be a welcome event. And with knowledge of herbs and other complementary therapies, menstrual regularity and natural abortion can usually be managed.

Acquiring complete information about one's body and cycle provides a basis of comparison and enables understanding of what is one's norm. You need all this information to have the right words to describe your own menstrual phases. Nan Koehler, a friend and midwife from California, puts it thus:

> *After several months you will be able to draw your own conclusions about what is normal for you and when your body deviates from this norm. This information is important in order to have a better understanding of your body. It will also be helpful when you decide to visit a medical doctor. Your will feel more confident about what is happening to you and you will be better equipped to make decisions concerning the type of medical care you want and need.*

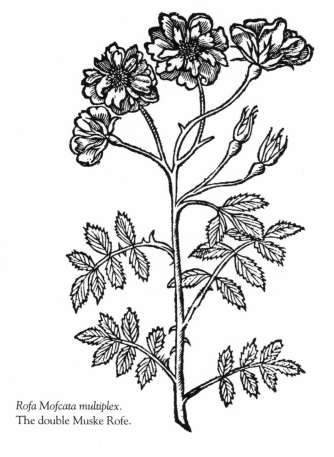

Rofa Mofcata multiplex.
The double Muske Rofe.

Chapter 4

Twelve Ways Not To Get Pregnant

By permission of Ruth Mayer
Adapted from Mademoiselle, *August 1993*

There's always abstinence. But barring that, which of these contraception methods gives the best deal—with the least risk,
cost, and hassle?

The Cervical Cap

What: Thimble-shaped rubber cap (user fills with spermicide)
that fits snugly over a thimble-shaped cervix. **How:** Prevents
sperm from entering uterus; spermicide renders sperm inactive.
Effectiveness: 80% to 98%. **Satisfaction:** N.A. **Plus:** Some
protection against pelvic inflammatory disease and certain sexually transmitted diseases. **Minus:** User should have normal Pap
test (can cause abnormal cell growth in cervix); some people
are allergic to rubber, spermicide; toxic shock syndrome (very
rare). **Caution:** Women with short fingers may have trouble
inserting the cap. **Cost/Prescription:** $13–25.

The Condom

At one time this author and several friends made a concerted
effort to collect all known types of condoms. We gave up at

about 200 and had great fun using these varicolored, multi-hued, many-shaped objects.

What: Latex or animal-tissue sheath placed over penis. **How:** Collects sperm so it doesn't enter uterus. **Effectiveness:** 64% to 97%. **Satisfaction:** 88% general. **Plus:** Latex (rather than animal skin) condoms are the best protection against AIDS and other sexually transmitted diseases; even better if used with the spermicide nonoxynol-9. **Minus:** Some people are allergic to latex. **Caution:** Don't use oil-based lubricants or essential oils with condoms—they can weaken the latex. **Cost/Over the counter:** $6–11.

The Diaphragm

We have also collected the various types of diaphragms and some types are easier to insert than others. Ask your doctor to describe and show you the different types.

What: Latex disk (user fills with spermicide) inserted to cover cervix. **How:** Prevents sperm from entering uterus; spermicide renders sperm inactive. **Effectiveness:** 80% to 98%. **Satisfaction:** 88% general. **Plus:** Some protection against pelvic inflammatory disease, sexually transmitted diseases; reduces risk of cervical cancer. **Minus:** Higher rate of urinary tract infections; some people are allergic to latex, spermicide; toxic shock syndrome (very rare). **Caution:** A women who gains or loses ten pounds should be refitted. **Cost/Prescription:** $13–25.

Spermicide

What: Foam, cream, gel, jelly, or suppository that contains a chemical agent (nonoxynol-9 or octoxynol). **How:** Kills or renders sperm inactive. **Effectiveness:** 70% to 80%. **Satisfaction:** N.A. **Plus:** Helps protect against some sexually transmitted diseases. **Minus:** Some people are allergic; more effective when used with diaphragm, condom, or cervical cap. **Caution:** Use just before intercourse; reapply every thirty minutes (effectiveness of some forms drops rapidly after a half hour). **Cost/Over the counter:** under $10 a tube.

The Sponge

What: Sponge of soft synthetic material containing spermicide; fits over cervix. **How:** Sponge prevents sperm from entering uterus; spermicide renders sperm inactive for twenty-four hours. **Effectiveness:** 80% to 87%. **Satisfaction:** 88% general. **Plus:** Some protection against certain sexually transmitted diseases. **Minus:** Irritation, allergic reaction, toxic shock syndrome (very rare). **Caution:** Must be moistened to activate spermicide; can be used repeatedly during 24-hour period, but must be left in for at least six hours after last intercourse. **Cost/Over the counter:** $3–5 for three.

Depo-Provera

What: Injection of synthetic hormone, progestin; good for three months. **How:** Prevents ovaries from releasing egg; alters chemistry, taste, and smell of cervical mucus and blocks sperm. **Effectiveness:** 99.6%. **Satisfaction:** N.A. **Plus:** May lessen risk of endometrial cancer; lighter periods or none at all (thus can prevent iron deficiency). **Minus:** May make oral intercourse unpleasant because of taste and smell changes; possible weight gain, headache, fatigue; risk for women who have had liver disease, unusual vaginal bleeding, breast cancer; may increase risk of osteoporosis, breast cancer; does not protect against sexually transmitted diseases. **Cost/Doctor visit:** $30 for three months.

The Pill

What: Combination of two synthetic hormones, estrogen and progestin. **How:** Prevents ovaries from releasing egg, alters cervical mucus to block sperm. **Effectiveness:** 99%. **Satisfaction:** 92% general. **Plus:** Less risk of pelvic inflammatory disease, ovarian and endometrial cancer; some protection against benign breast tumors and ovarian cysts. **Minus:** Nausea, depression; increased risk for women who smoke or have had blood clots, heart attack, stroke, liver tumor; does not protect against sexually transmitted diseases. **Cost/Prescription:** $10–30 per month.

The Mini Pill

What: Contains one synthetic hormone, progestin, in lower dose than the Pill. **How:** Alters cervical mucus to block sperm or prevents fertilized egg from implanting in uterus. **Effectiveness:** 97%. **Satisfaction:** N.A. **Plus:** Doesn't contain estrogen, so no added risk of blood clots, heart attack, or stroke. **Minus:** Spotting between periods; does not protect against sexually transmitted diseases. **Caution:** If the Mini Pill is missed for even one day, it is unreliable for the rest of the month; also, it is more effective if taken at the same time every day. **Cost/Prescription:** $10–30 per month.

The IUD

What: IntraUterine (i.e., inside womb) Device that contains copper (ParaGuard Copper; good for eight years) or releases a hormone (Progestasert; good for one year). **How:** Prevents fertilization of egg or changes uterine lining so fertilized egg can't implant. **Effectiveness:** 97% general. **Satisfaction:** 98%. **Plus:** None. **Minus:** Higher risk of pelvic infection; risk of sterility or puncture of uterus (very rare); if pregnancy occurs while IUD is in place, miscarriage or ectopic (outside-the-uterus) pregnancy more likely. **Cost/Doctor visit:** $140 and up.

Implants (Norplant)

What: Six matchstick-size inserts under skin of upper arm; good for five years. **How:** Releases synthetic hormone (levonorgestrel) that prevents ovulation; alters cervical mucus to block sperm. **Effectiveness:** 99%. **Satisfaction:** N.A. **Plus:** Lighter periods;

contains no estrogen, so no added risk of blood clots. **Minus:** Periods may become irregular or stop; possible depression, headache, nausea, loss of appetite, enlarged ovaries, weight gain, growth of body/facial hair, breast tenderness. **Cost/Doctor visit:** $500–600.

Female Sterilization

What: Fallopian tubes are cut or clamped. **How:** Prevents eggs from traveling from ovaries to uterus. **Effectiveness:** 99% when cut. **Satisfaction:** 90% general. **Plus:** None. Minus: Risk of surgical complication or reaction to general anesthetic; postsurgical pain/discomfort; may increase risk of later hysterectomy; does not protect against sexually transmitted diseases. **Caution:** If procedure is misperformed, pregnancy could occur (very rare). **Cost/Surgery:** $1,000–2,500. This procedure can occasionally be undone.

Future Contraceptives

For Women

- A **female condom** (brand name: *Reality*) was approved by the Food and Drug Administration (FDA) in April 1993, but hasn't been out long enough to yield statistics. It's a polyurethane sheath that lines the vagina; like the male condom, it helps protect—but is less effective—against sexually transmitted diseases, including AIDS.

- A **contraceptive ring** is a doughnut-shaped device that's inserted into the vagina, where it releases pregnancy-preventing hormones. Two types are now in FDA-approved clinical trials.

- The **improved implant** (brand name: *Norplant II*), with two rods rather than six, would be easier to insert and remove. Currently seeking approval for FDA-sanctioned clinical trials.

- **Lea's Shield** is a cup-shaped bowl that covers the cervix; it's said to fit particularly well and would be sold without a prescription. Currently in FDA-approved clinical trials.

- **Fem Cap** is a hypoallergenic silicone* and rubber cap; its "brim" is supposed to provide a more secure fit and an airtight seal over the cervix. Smaller than a diaphragm, it's also said to be less noticeable during intercourse. It would come in three sizes and require a prescription. Currently in FDA-approved clinical trials.

*Silicone can cause immune system deficiency.

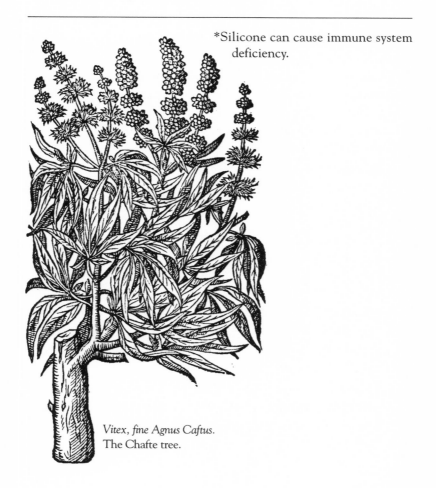

Vitex, fine Agnus Caftus.
The Chafte tree.

Chapter 5

Herbs for Females

There are dozens of plants that aid the reproductive organs and regulate a woman's cycle. Many plants are known for their estrogenic activity[2] and others such as ***Vitex Agnus Castus***[3,4] relieve premenstrual water retention, menstrual problems, and even the acne associated with hormonal changes. ***Vitex Agnus Castus*** is not well known in the United States but is well known and well documented in other countries.

   Black Cohosh and **Blue Cohosh** were used by Native Americans and are thought to help overcome pathological conditions in the reproductive organs. These two have a powerful action on the central nervous system. **Black Cohosh** prepares the uterus for birth, makes labor less difficult, and relieves uterine distress during the actual birthing. **Black Cohosh** is often used with **Raspberry leaves,** and works best when drunk daily throughout pregnancy. **Blue Cohosh** is used after childbirth or to prolong the pregnancy until the fetus is properly developed. It is often used as a tea with **Raspberry leaf** from the sixth month of pregnancy until the last two weeks when **Black Cohosh** is substituted. **Blue Cohosh** is considered to be a preventive of miscarriage.

   Black Horehound is used mainly for the respiratory system for continuous coughs but has also been used as a calmative for

hysteria and as a uterine tonic. **Black Willow** is an anaphrodisiac and a sedative tonic for the reproductive organs. **Burdock
seed** is mainly used for skin care as a cosmetic wash and **Burdock root** is used internally in all blood-purifying mixtures
because it has an alterative, diuretic, and astringent action. It
also has a great healing influence on the sebaceous and sweat
glands and is used for uterine displacements. In this latter case
it is added to the Basic Bolus Formula.

Cowslip has been used as a tea and a douche for uterine
tumors, and as a mild sedative.

Marjoram herb, a mild sedative, is also used for certain uterine tumors and helps to regulate the cycle when used as a douche
because it acts as an emmenagogue (to bring on the menses). It
is a warming herb: the tea is drunk to help ease an asthma attack,
and the infused oil is good for rubbing stiff limbs (especially
when a few drops of **essential oil of Rosemary** are added). The
herb can also be used in baths as a mild stimulant. **Motherwort**
is tonic, nervine, and an emmenagogue, and it has a soothing,
relaxing effect on the heart and the uterus, seeming to relieve
nervous disorders in both these organs. **Myrtle leaves (*Myrtus
communis*),** also a nerve sedative, stimulates the mucous secretions of the vagina and is therefore helpful to older women (past
menopause) whose lack of estrogen diminishes the vaginal lubricants. **Myrtle leaf** is best either as a tea used as a douche or
drunk as a beverage. It can be deliciously aromatic, an excellent vaginal douche on the last day of the menses. I like to call
Mugwort "the young girl's herb" because it helps relieve the
cramps that often accompany a pubescent girl's first few periods. **Mugwort** taken as a beverage tea, one cup per day for a few
months, also helps regulate the cycle.

Pennyroyal tops are considered by the great English herbalist Hilda Leyel to be an herb specific for the left side, the left
kidney, the left ureter, and/or the reproductive organs and the

Achilles tendon. Taken in *small* doses* this herb tea helps regulate the cycle and soothe spasmodic contractions of the uterus.
Taken in larger doses it can be part of a program for "natural"
abortion. It is unknown at this time if using *very* large amounts
of **Pennyroyal tea** can harm a fetus (the essential oil <u>IS</u> harmful).

Wild Thyme, a mild sedative and an antiseptic astringent,
is used for nervous disorders that arise from any problem in the
reproductive organs.

These are some of the herbs that have been used for the
reproductive system of women. They are not difficult to use.
Herbalists, especially we women herbalists, should take charge
of our health. We should use herbs as our allies, "a helpful friend,"
and take them along with other good health measures. These
other measures include a wholesome and unprocessed diet, exercise, moderate living, nutritional supplements, and, of course,
the herbs to relieve some of the so-called "normal" miseries of
womanhood.

It is not, however, "normal" to have heavy menstrual discharge or to lack the menses altogether. It is not "normal" to
have extremely painful childbirth or to lack milk for one's newborn. Women can have menstrual regularity, natural abortions,
and relatively painless childbirth—all this using herbs. These
things take only minimal knowledge of plant use. But do not
expect to take an herb tea for a few days to undo ten years of
poor habits; do not expect to take a few herbal capsules just prior
to birth to ensure a normal delivery. Herbal medicine requires
a lifetime of moderation, eating a wholesome diet of fresh,
unprocessed foods, and exercising the body with regularity. There
are no cure-alls for a lifetime of dissipations. Moderation in
habits, good nutrition, regular exercise, clear air, and pure water

---

*One tsp/cup water, steep three minutes, strain. Drink one cup/day.

to drink work hand in hand with an herbal regime to ensure a healthy recovery from whatever ails you.

Each woman is different, having a unique cultural and genetic background. Herbal formulations should be designed individually to take into consideration these differences. When one herbal mixture fails, a competent herbalist can design another that will work. Here is the fundamental difference between the herbalist and the doctor: with his limited pharmacopoeial background, an allopathic doctor (MD) prescribes a general formula that works in most of his/her cases. An herbalist composes an herbal formula for the case that is current, taking into consideration various factors, such as food habits, lifestyle, etc.

Individual herbs have occasionally been "scientifically" studied, their medicinal value qualitatively and quantitatively determined. But in most cases we use herbs that have been known and used for thousands of years but have not necessarily been given the medical "stamp of approval" by investigative scientists. We "know" that these formulas work because women, as herb-doctors, have used them with great success for thousands of years.

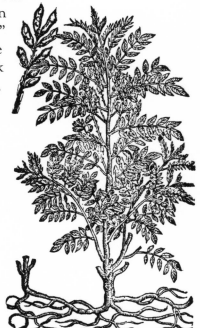

Glycyrrhiza vulgaris.
Common Licorice.

Chapter 6

Herbal Formulas for Women
From Menarch to Menopause

Menstrual Tardiness (especially when pregnancy is to be avoided). It is unfortunate that the medical profession has not examined the various herbal alternatives to surgery in terminating a pregnancy or simply in establishing regularity in the menstrual cycle. The methods recommended here have not to my knowledge been closely examined, but for many women these methods have worked with great success, *when used together.* A woman ought to know when her menses is due. If the menstrual cycle is expected to be late, several combinations of plants can be used.

1. **Apricot kernels,** suspected to have anticancer qualities, possibly prevent implantation by treating the developing fetus as just another foreign body. Take them eight at a time, three times a day, from ovulation until day one of the menstrual cycle (when bleeding first occurs). They have to be finely chopped or carefully chewed. (Of course, it is easier to purchase the kernels than to try to extract them from the Apricot pit.)

2. **Parsley,** freshly washed and clean, may be wadded up into the shape of a tampon and inserted into the vagina three days before the period is due. This herbal plug is left for

24–36 hours before it is removed and replaced with a fresh sprig. It will collect mucus and can develop a rather strong odor. The Parsley can be replaced as often as necessary (every half-day) until the period is well established.

3. **Carrot seeds** can be ingested from ovulation to the end of the cycle to inhibit the egg from implanting on the uterine wall and to ensure that the menses will begin. They can be used as an abortive even after the period has been missed. Scientific investigation has shown **Carrot oil** from the seeds to be a direct cardiac depressant[5] and to have a relaxing effect on the uterus of some mammals. Possibly this relaxing effect is the reason it has been effective as an abortive (inhibiting implantation) in women.

4. A lovely flower, the **Evening Primrose,** has been the source of a fluid extract used by women prior to labor or as an abortive. Formerly the fluid extract (infusion) was ingested as well as used as a vaginal douche. The seed oil contains gamma linolenic acid and linoleic acid, precursors to prostaglandin production in the body. A high level of prostaglandin softens the cervix to prepare it for expansion during labor. Now we use the **Oil of Evening Primrose** seed capsules, three times per day from ovulation until the period is due, to ensure the menses if birth control measures have been lax. The oil can also be directly applied to the cervix several times a day just before the period is due.

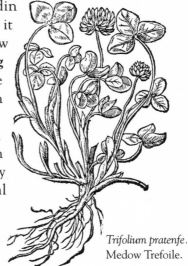

Trifolium pratenfe.
Medow Trefoile.

5. **Pennyroyal tea** (*not* oil of Pennyroyal) is taken a quart a day, for not more than four days beginning on the day before the period is due and until day four if the period is late. Make the (tea) infusion by taking ½ to 1 pound of the dried herb and adding to it 4–6 quarts of hot water. Allow the herb to steep in the water for at least 24 hours, then strain. Drink the tea, half a cup at a time, every waking hour, for four days.*

6. **Vitamin C** in large amounts also seems to encourage the release of the uterine lining. Ten to fifteen (10–15) grams can be taken daily, at intervals throughout the day, from ovulation until menses to ensure a menstrual flow.

7. **Diet** is very important when there is a suspected pregnancy or when a woman wishes to establish menstrual regularity. A 70 to 80% fresh, raw, or steamed alkaline-forming diet is encouraged. This diet allows vegetables, fruits, Potatoes of all kinds, Millet as a grain, and Almonds as the nut, while limiting other grains, nuts, and meats to 20 to 30% by weight of the diet. Just before a woman's period she should eat lightly of whole foods and drink plenty of water, herb teas, and vegetable juices.

8. Lastly, **exercise** vigorously as constantly as possible until the menses is well established.

These eight steps, combined, "bring on" the period when it is late, for whatever the reason. Steps 2, 7, and 8 also establish regularity, along with the teas discussed next.

---

*In the 1970s, a woman committed suicide by ingesting half an ounce of Pennyroyal oil. It slowly and painfully destroyed her liver. The oil, like all essential oils, is a deadly poison when taken in large amounts. And a large amount is anything over 1–2 drops at a time, more than once a day.

Menarche*

Menarche is that time in a girl's life when she has her first menstrual cycle. It occurs earlier and earlier these days, sometimes to girls as young as nine years old. But it always occurs very soon after the girl reaches a weight of ninety-two to 102 pounds. For small girls or young women who exercise heavily, such as gymnasts, the menarche may not occur until the early teens.

I remember my own early menstrual cycles. They were extensive and I bled heavily. At the time I was a swimmer, and during the summer when I was swimming these periods would lighten up considerably. In any case, I was twelve-and-a-half and by the time I was thirteen, my periods evolved into three- to five-day events every twenty-five days. My daughter and her friends had a similar cycle. The herbs that we used were simple herbs, easily used and taken in teas or by capsules.

Herbal teas should be taken daily and include high-calcium herbs such as **Borage flowers** and **leaves,** small amounts of **Angelica root** or **Dong Quai root** which will balance the hormonal system, **Parsley leaf** for the cleansing effect of chlorophyll, and **Echinacea root** for its antiseptic qualities and as a "blood cleanser." This mixture of equal parts of the herbs and roots taken as an infusion daily will ease excess bleeding and act to treat the skin as well and free it from acne and pimples. The young girl (and even young boys will benefit) should take one to two cups per day of this tea.

Body odor can be treated with the inclusion of edible clay in the diet. One teaspoon added to one-half glass of water is drunk every night before bed followed by a full glass of water.

---

*For more information, please read "The Herbal Child," Chapter 4 of *Jeanne Rose's Modern Herbal,* published by Perigee Books. Available for $10.95 + $1.50 shipping from the Herbal Studies Library. See Source List, p. 121.

A child going through puberty often has bad body odor that no amount of bathing can cure. The addition of clay is very helpful and to my personal knowledge is 100% effective in taking care of this problem which results from new hormones coursing through the body, the addition of weight and size, and added bone growth. The edible clays that are available on the market are tasteless; they adsorb toxins and are excreted with the feces in the morning. Green clay and edible clays are available through most health food stores or from Mountain Rose Herbs in Redway, CA, or Phybiosis in Bowie, MD. See Source List, pp. 123–124.

Aromatherapy for the Menarche

The essential oils can be used by inhalation or by application in massage oils to treat early periods, excessive periods, and scanty or late periods.

For excessive bleeding (menorrhagia) use **Rose** oil by massage and inhalation. For irregular periods use daily applications of **Clary Sage** oil or **Rose** oil and *inhale* **Clary Sage** oil regularly using a hankie or diffusor. For painful periods use *applications* of the essential oils of **Anise seed, Carrot seed, Jasmine,** and **Rose** and *inhale* the essential oils of **Clary Sage** and **Rose.** For scanty or late periods (amenorrhea) *apply* the essential oils of **Fennel seed,** true **Lavender,** and **Rosemary** and *inhale* the essential oils of **Clary Sage** for balance, **Fennel seed** for hormonal balance, and **Jasmine,** true **Lavender,** or **Roman Chamomile** oils for emotional balance and to dispel depression.

The massage oil may be made with the same herbs by infusion (1 oz mixed herbs to 1 quart Olive oil) and then their essential oils added, 10–20 drops of essential oil to every ounce of massage oil. Massage in a gentle rotary motion the area below the diaphragm and down to the upper thighs. The lower back can also be massaged as it will include the first chakra which lies within and controls the reproductive organs.

Don't forget when treating the young person that other factors should be weighed, including complete nutrition, vitamins and minerals, clean water, and the *reduction* or avoidance of hormone-laced foods such as meats and pesticide-sprayed fruits and vegetables. Get your food from certified organic sources.

Menstrual Regulation

It has long been known that estrogens naturally occur in certain plant foods[2,6] as well as in certain medicinal herbs. **Licorice root** and **Angelica** have been carefully examined and found to be characterized by considerable amounts of plant estrogens.[7,8] In addition, **Licorice root** when given in large amounts has caused premature sex maturation in young animals.[9] Herbalists use **Licorice** and **Red Clover**[10]* in the estrogen phase of the menstrual cycle and then **Sarsaparilla** and **Blessed Thistle** for their progesterone type content in the progesterone phase. *Vitex Agnus Castus* is thought to benefit the pituitary, balancing hormone production.

Estrogen Tea— from Day 1 to 10	Progesterone Tea— from Days 10 to 27
Licorice root[26]—1 part	**Sarsaparilla root**—4 parts
Angelica root—1 part	**Blessed Thistle**—2 parts
Peony root[26]—1 part	**Raspberry leaf**—4 parts
Agnus Castus—1 part	**Ginseng root**—1 part
Red Clover tops—1 part	**Agnus Castus seed**—1 part

The infusion is made in the standard way: 1 ounce of the dried mixed herbs is steeped (infused) in 1 quart of water just

*Red Clover has been shown to induce sterility when eaten in large amounts by forage animals. In smaller amounts it stimulates reproductive function because of its phyto-estrogenic content. Can drinking large amounts of Red Clover tea daily induce temporary sterility in women? And what effect would this ultimately have on her uterus?

under the boiling point for at least twenty minutes. Strain out the herbs and drink the liquid, 6 ounces of it, three times per day, during the days indicated.

On days 27, 28, and day 1, or the comparable days when the cycle is normally longer or shorter, the **Parsley** insertion and the dietary advice outlined in steps 2, 7, and 8 (pp. 23–24, 25) are recommended. Dian Buchman, an herbalist, recommends eating **Carrots** every day to regulate the menstrual cycle.

Premenstrual Tension, Acne, and Water Retention

For this condition, I recommend a light diet deleting all refined foods, sugar, alcohol, and stimulants. Take a tea of **Vitex Agnus Castus seeds** with **Rosemary herb** (for its tonic effect) several times a day for several days just prior to the menses. **Vitex Agnus Castus** has been shown to relieve premenstrual water retention[3] as well as several forms of acne. Supplements such as potassium, calcium in the form of bone meal, and vitamins C and B_6 are also helpful.

Vaginal Infections

These methods can be used for all vaginal infections, regardless of source.

• PID (Pelvic Inflammatory Disease)

Most forms of vaginal infection, including PID, Gardnerella (*Hemophilus*), fungus, yeast, and bacteria, respond to two herbal treatments—an herbal bolus inserted into the vagina and herbal capsules taken by mouth. The herbal capsules consist of a basic formula of **Yellow Dock root** to cleanse the blood, **Echinacea root** to fight infection by encouraging the production of white blood cells, **Golden Seal root** to counteract bacteria and viruses, and **Ginseng root** to encourage the health of the lymphatic system. This is called the **YEGG Formula.**™

The bolus should include the herbs that are in the capsules as well as **Slippery Elm bark, Comfrey root,** and **Marshmallow root.** The bolus herbs should be powdered and mixed with enough melted cocoa butter to hold the mass together, and a piece one-half inch in diameter and one inch long can be inserted high in the vagina every thirty-six hours. It can be held in place with a tampon. Douche it out at the end of thirty-six hours with an infusion of an herbal mixture of **Yellow Dock, Golden Seal,** and **Comfrey root.** Use this bolus and douche for six days, rest one day, then repeat at least twice more for a total of three to six weeks or until the infection completely clears up.

These formulas and the method will be repeated again in greater detail on later pages. These formulas also require the same diet, exercise, and supplements as for menstrual tardiness. The bolus, by the way, plays hell with your sex life; it is not too tidy to have intercourse with a wad of herbs in your vagina.

• Yeast infections

Specific recommendations for various vaginal disorders include Yogurt as a douche for yeast infections—or apply it with a standard contraceptive cream applicator. You can use plain vinegar and water as a douche to reestablish the normal acidity of the vagina. This is also effective for Trichomonas and Gardnerella (*Hemophilus vaginalis*).

The medicinal aspects of **Garlic**[11] have been extensively studied and shown to have antiviral, antibacterial,[12,13] antifungal,[14] and pesticidal properties. Trichomonas, a protozoan, can be treated with **Garlic** suppositories. Wrap a small piece of **Garlic** (a small clove) in thin cheesecloth or just use it as is* and insert it into the vagina. Replace the **Garlic** every twelve hours until the infection clears up. **Garlic** (4 finely chopped cloves per ½

---

*Sometimes cheesecloth leaves little fibers in the vagina that can cause irritation.

cup yogurt) can also be infused (soaked or steeped) in plain yogurt for several days, strained out, and the yogurt inserted into the vagina with a vaginal applicator.

• Bacterial Infections

Bacterial infections, including Gardnerella (*Hemophilus*) or PID, are best treated with the herbal capsules and the bolus. PID (Pelvic Inflammatory Disease) is one of the most difficult illnesses to diagnose and treat. One woman I'm acquainted with has been off and on antibiotics for three years with no relief from her pain and discomfort. PID is often a result of the migration of intestinal bacteria into the reproductive tract. Gardnerella (previously called *Hemophilus vaginalis*) is often the culprit. Even now, physicians call this bacteria a Hemophilus when it inhabits the vagina causing vaginitis, and Gardnerella when it lives where it is supposed to, in the intestine. When it migrates into the uterus it is often diagnosed as "PID" generally, of unknown origin.

Bacterias produce gas as a by-product. When this gas is in the uterus it can cause a great deal of pain and suffering. Bacterial infections in the vagina are also called nonspecific vaginitis and usually produce a heavy, irritating, itchy, smelly discharge that may be yellow to greenish-yellow and quite profuse and runny. An herbal vinegar and water douche taken once or twice a day for a few days may be all that is necessary to kill off a bacterial infection such as this, or you may wish to use one of the other remedies already described.

Chlamydia is an infection in the cervical cells. Generally, home remedies are considered not worthy for this infection, but the **YEGG Formula** should be used since it detoxifies the uterus.

But back to **PID** of the uterus. PID may be a result of a new love affair when all too much time is spent in bed exploring various positions and making love sequentially without bathing between bouts of intercourse. This happened to me, while renew-

ing a relationship with an ex-lover after an extensive trip to the
Bahamas and into Mexico. I got violently sick, vomited, had
diarrhea, intense abdominal cramps, then a bout of constipa-
tion. I took to my bed. This pain and sickness was so unlike my
body's usual behavior that I fasted, consulted all my healer friends,
undertook a cleansing ritual by an herbalist trained in India,
drank **Carrot** juice for a week, and took **Chlorella** and lactobacillus tablets in the vain hope this would cure me. At this
point I thought I was suffering from a bacterial infection of the
intestines that I might have picked up in Mexico. If I'd had any
sense I would have used my famous wonder **YEGG Formula** of
Yellow Dock root, Echinacea root, Golden Seal root, and **Ginseng root.** But even herbalists forget their knowledge when it
comes to treating themselves.* I panicked, and forgot everything I knew.

Finally, some two months after my Mexico trip and having
spent four out of eight weeks in bed, I consulted a physician.
He took stool samples for parasites, turned me upside down for
a proctosigmoidoscopy (a tube inserted in the anus to examine
the walls of the large intestine for irregularities), felt around my
uterus, and declared in an extremely serious voice that my uterus
was grossly enlarged and should be removed immediately. I had
spent most of the previous time with an altered consciousness
from taking pain pills and drinking tequila in the vain hope that
the Mexican bacteria would get drunk on their native juice and
die a happy death.

This diagnosis was so terrifying that I immediately wrote a
will, informed my family and friends of the deposition of certain items I wanted them to have, and wrote all my long-over-
due letters. I then made an appointment with another doctor
for a second opinion. After a series of blood and urine tests, he

---

*Who was it that said, "A healer who treats himself has a fool for a
patient"?

declared that I was dehydrated and that my uterus had a large cyst, was probably diseased, and should be immediately removed.

At this point I consulted a psychic, who told me there was a problem in my uterus but not as serious as the doctors had led me to believe. I started a color cure, a regime guaranteed by an East Indian man to cure cysts and tumors of the uterus. I also made an appointment (the third) with the OB/Gyn who had delivered my son nine years before and was no doubt familiar with the idiosyncrasies of my uterus. I had to wait five days for the appointment and spent the time doing color-scented baths, eating **Melons,** and drinking **Carrot juice.** This doctor took one look at my enlarged belly, palpated my painfully tender uterus, and wisely took a scraping of vaginal walls and drippings from the cervix which he examined under the microscope. "My, you must have been in a great deal of pain lately," he said. I agreed. He then said that it was a *simple* infection caused by Gardnerella, that I should abstain from intercourse (which I had been unable to participate in anyway because of the pain), drink plenty of water, and take Ampicillin for five days. As an herbalist I have a strong dislike of antibiotics, but I weighed my aversion against my desire to get well (instantaneously and deal with the side effects later), and took the prescription.

After three days on the Ampicillin the pain began to subside. After five days it came back and put me to bed again. The OB/Gyn advised me to admit myself into the hospital and to be put on antibiotics intravenously (at least until he found the correct antibiotic — or "tics" — to kill *my* bacteria). At this time, I wondered why a culture of my "little beasties" (that is, the creatures that were causing the infection) had not already been grown in the lab, so that the antibiotic that was prescribed would be the proper one to kill my particular bacteria. Wondering why a culture grown in the laboratory would not have worked just as well as using *me* as a test subject in the hospital, I balked and absolutely refused to be hospitalized. Finally, common sense and knowledge came back into my pain-addled head and I began to take my own special remedies. Within *three* days of taking the YEGG Formula, I was out of pain. In five days my belly subsided to a more fashionable flattened appearance. Within seven days, I was my old healthy happy self again.

What does all this prove?

1. No matter what the condition—skin, prostate, uterus, intestine, or infection—**TAKE THE YEGG Formula** — three capsules three times per day for at least nine days. (See next page.)

2. Always **get a second opinion** and *even a third* before believing a diagnosis that includes surgery and certainly before submitting to surgery.

3. **Herbs work.** Sometimes slowly, sometimes quickly, but they do "cure" (most certainly). However, you may have to alter your lifestyle to get the most benefits from the herbs that have been prescribed for your particular problem.

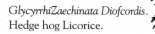

GlycyrrhiZaechinata Diofcordis.
Hedge hog Licorice.

The Basic YEGG Formula

For Any Uterine or Vaginal Infection

> 1 oz powdered **Yellow Dock root**
> 2 oz powdered **Echinacea root**
> 1 oz powdered **Golden Seal root**
> 1 oz powdered **Ginseng or Ginger root** (Ginseng for
> the lymphatic system or Ginger for the digestive or
> eliminatory system)

Mix together the dry, powdered herbs and stuff them into size 00 gelatin capsules. There is a marvelous gadget called Cap · M· Quick that takes size 00 capsules—fifty at a time, i.e., usually a five-day supply—and fills the fifty caps in about five minutes.

The Basic YEGG Formula should be taken for about ten days, three capsules three times per day just prior to or just after a meal.

The Basic Formula for a Bolus

> ½ oz each of the following herbs, dried and powdered:
> **Yellow Dock root, Echinacea root, Squaw Vine,**
> **Golden Seal root, Slippery Elm bark, Chickweed,**
> **Comfrey root, Marshmallow root**
> One handful finely chopped fresh **Chickweed,** if
> possible.

Mix together all the herbs and add melted Cocoa butter until the mass just holds together—about 2½ oz herbs to ½ cup melted Cocoa butter. Use a sheet of wax paper to roll out the mixture into a slim sausage shape. Roll until you get a uniform, long, slim sausage about ½ inch in diameter. Refrigerate or freeze until hard. Cut into one-inch pieces and freeze again until needed. Use as directed for six weeks to six months.

An even easier "Bolus" is a gelatin capsule of Garlic infused oil. Insert high in the vagina 1x/day (or 2x/day if infection is bad) until all symptoms are gone. Use pure (no chemical) yogurt for symptom relief externally. Many herbalists consider douching not a good practice.

The Basic Formula for a Cleansing Douche

> ½ oz each of the following herbs, dried (but not powdered) and cut: **Yellow Dock, Golden Seal, Comfrey root.**
> 1 quart of water

Bring all ingredients to a boil and simmer for twenty minutes. Cool, strain, and use. Makes three treatments.

Aromatherapy Treatments for Uterine and Vaginal Infections

There are many essential oils that can be used for vaginal infections and inflammations. The oils are used in douches, sitz baths, via application on a tampon and inserted, in creams and ointments, and in lotions used for massage. For internal infections using essential oils by inhalation only works to ease stress and tension and allay fears of consequence.

The favorite and safest essential oils to use are true **Lavender** and **Tea Tree** and occasionally **Clary Sage** and **German Chamomile.** Almost all infections including leucorrhea, trichomonas, nonspecific vaginitis, and Gardnerella, which is a bacterial infection often causing PID, can be treated with essential oils.

The essential oil needs to be diluted slightly either in yogurt or vinegar if the vagina is too alkaline, or with pure water and vegetable glycerine or baking soda solution if the vagina is too acid or very irritated. Generally, 2 drops of essential oil are diluted in ½ cup of the carrier substance and applied.

• Tampon

> 2 drops essential oil (**Tea Tree** and/or true **Lavender**)
> ½ cup carrier substance

Soak a tampon in this and insert, using a new tampon every twelve hours. Use for a week.

• Vinegar or Yogurt Douche

> 8 drops essential oil (**Tea Tree** and/or true **Lavender**)

Add these to ¼ cup vinegar or ½ cup yogurt. Shake carefully and then dilute with 1 cup body-temperature spring water and douche at least once per day for three days using other methods as necessary. We all know that douching upsets the normal acid/ alkaline balance of the vagina, so use douching only on an emergency basis and not as a daily routine.

• Creams, Lotions, and Ointments

These can be applied by gentle massage or simple application to the irritated tissues. Take a plain unscented cream, simple Olive or Jojoba oil, or any simple unscented lotion, and add a total of 20 drops of essential oil (**Tea tree** and true **Lavender**) to each ounce, and apply twice a day. It pays to make only one ounce at a time as various oils and combinations can be experimented with until the correct one is found for your particular case. An ounce of essential oil in cream, lotion, or oil will last for quite a bit of time, even several weeks, as only a few drops are used at any one time.

• Sitz Baths

Sitz baths are an old-fashioned means to treat irritated vaginal and labial tissue, but a very effective one. Take 8–10 drops or more of your essential oil mixture and add to 1 quart of body-temperature water and you sit in this for twenty minutes twice a day. If you don't have a pot big enough and shallow enough to sit in, you can also add two inches of body-temperature water to your bath tub and sit in that, although I suggest you wrap your shoulders with a towel so that your upper body does not get chilled.

Once, many years ago, I had an outdoor tub under a spreading wild **Lilac** bush, and when I needed a simple sitz bath, I would half-fill the tub with hot water, add herbs picked on the way to the tub, and then add a few drops of **Peppermint oil** that I then swirled in. At that time I did not know about **Tea Tree oil** and **Peppermint** was all I had. This combination of herbs and essential oil worked great. The herbs were **Comfrey, Sage,** and wild **Mint.**

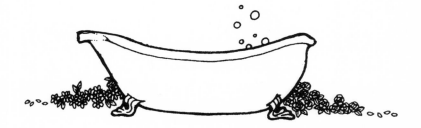

Bladder and Kidney Infections

UTI (Urinary Tract Infections), Cystitis

(See Herbs for Urinary System, Herbal Studies Course, Chapter 22.)

Cystitis (bacterial infections in the bladder) may occur in women through intercourse or childbirth or as a result of using standard medicinal drugs prescribed for vaginitis. Cystitis can be easily cured at home by using the recommended diet already mentioned, drinking 1 quart per day of unsweetened **Cranberry juice,** and taking (up to) 10 grams of vitamin C per day. The juice and the C (the latter two ingredients) act as antiseptics in the bladder and they also sterilize the urine. Any of the herbs mentioned for cystitis can be soaked (infused) in the **Cranberry juice** to increase its effectiveness, and these herbs can also be taken in as a standard infusion/tea throughout the day. In addition, when cystitis results from strenuous intercourse, check the vulva for external cuts or bruises. These can be treated with sitz baths of **Comfrey root.** Urinate both before and after intercourse to flush out whatever bacteria may be lurking in the bladder and remember also to drink plenty of water or herb tea throughout the day.

A Good Herbal Formula for Cystitis

2 oz **Uva-ursi leaves**	1 oz **Buchu leaves**
1 oz **Couch grass**	1 oz **Parsley root**
1 oz **Marshmallow root**	1 oz **Comfrey root**
½ oz **Juniper berries**	½ oz **Golden Seal root**
½ oz **Echinacea root**	

Mix the dried herbs together and make the infusion in the standard way, using ½ oz herbs to 1 quart of water.

Drink the strained infusion, one-half cup at half-hour intervals throughout the day until the quart of tea/infusion is gone.

Do this for at least five days and preferably until three days after the infection clears up.

Folia Uva-ursi (family *Ericaceae*), also called **Uva-ursi leaves,** is an official drug in the world pharmacopoeia. Its medicinal activity is due to arbutin and anthocyanins. Arbutin passes through the body unchanged, then hydrolyzes in the urine, but only if harmful bacteria are present. It then converts to hydro-quinone, becoming a disinfectant.[17] Anthocyanins possess a great affinity for certain tissues such as kidneys and skin; they increase capillary resistance and decrease capillary permeabil-ity.[16,18]

There are other species in the *Ericaceae* family such as **Huck-leberry** and **Blueberry** that actually contain more of the arbutin and anthocyanins than **Uva-ursi.** But **Uva-ursi** is more fre-quently used, probably because it is better known than its cousins and because it has been used more often for a longer period of time.

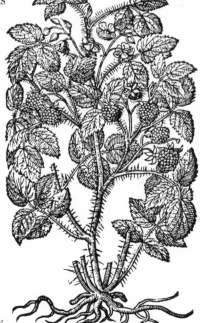

Rubus Idaus.
The Rafpis Bufh or Hinde-berry.

A Dietary Plan and Supplements
For Fibroid Tumors of the Uterus and Breast Cysts

No Drugs

No Alcohol during acute phase, moderate use of alcohol thereafter

No Nicotine

No Caffeine *ever*, including Black Tea, Chocolate, Coffee, Maté, Guarana

YEGG Formula (2:2:1:1 Ginseng)

Breakfast

Proteins such as eggs, wheat germ, whole grains.

SUPPLEMENTS:
    3–5 brewer's yeast tablets
    3–5 liver tablets
    2 antioxidants (Selenium, E, C)
    2 B-complex
    2 multi-minerals
    2–3 herbal menopause tablets
    10,000 units vitamin A
    SOD
    3 size 00 YEGG capsules

Lunch

Proteins such as seafoods, whole grains, steamed vegetables, wheat germ, soups, Sunflower seeds, Soy proteins.

SUPPLEMENTS:
    3–5 brewer's yeast tablets
    3–5 liver tablets
    2 antioxidants (Selenium, E, C)
    2 B-complex
    2 grams vitamin C
    2 multi-minerals
    2–3 herbal menopause tablets

SOD
500 mg inositol + 1000 mg choline
4 Apricot kernels
3 size 00 YEGG capsules

Dinner

Vegetables and salad with wheat germ, dressed in Olive oil
and Lemon juice and lots of herbs, and steamed or baked
Potatoes.

SUPPLEMENTS: 3–5 brewer's yeast tablets
                    3–5 liver tablets
                    2 antioxidants (Selenium, E, C)
                    2 B-complex
                    2 grams vitamin C
                    2 multi-minerals
                    2–3 herbal menopause tablets
                    SOD
                    2 size 00 YEGG capsules

Bedtime

SUPPLEMENTS: 3 brewer's yeast tablets
                    3 liver tablets
                    2 calcium magnesium tablets
                    50 mg B_6
                    800 units vitamin E
                    2 grams vitamin C
                    50–100 mg zinc
                    2–00 YEGG
                    3–5 Red Clover/Chapparal/
                        Gotu Kola tablets
                    10,000 vitamin A
                    SOD
                    8 Apricot kernels

- Fruits should be eaten upon waking up, any time throughout the day, or at bedtime, but not with other meals.

- The best vegetables are Asparagus, Beets, Cauliflower, Broccoli, Watercress, Garlic, Onion, Brussels sprouts, Lima beans, and Carrots.

- Juices should be fresh-squeezed, especially Carrot/Celery and Apple/Orange.

- SOD—sulfoxide dismutase. You may find it under other spellings in health food stores.

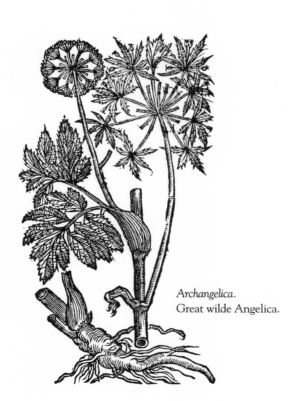

Archangelica.
Great wilde Angelica.

Chapter 7

Colortherapy

The use of color to treat conditions. A strange, obscure method of treatment.

The Color Cure for All Uterine Problems, Cysts, and Tumors:

PID, Uterine Cysts, and Tumor Remedies

1. **Oil:** Vigorous massage with *red* and *green* color-treated Olive oil. (Put some Olive oil in a green glass bottle and some in a red glass bottle, or wrap each bottle with silk of the appropriate color. Expose the "now-colored" bottles to the Sun for forty days.)*

   When you are ready to use the oils, mix together one ounce of each (i.e., green and red color-treated), put a bit of the oil on a piece of cotton, and rub the abdomen vigorously at least three times per day.

2. **Sun:** For color treatments in the Sun, alternate red and

---

*Obviously you must have color-treated Olive oil and water on hand all the time or else you may have to wait more than a month to treat yourself if you are diagnosed as having a tumor or cyst that needs to be removed. So the question arises—How long can it be stored and still be effective?

green light for ten minutes each day, one minute for each color. You may accomplish this in any of three ways: Place a piece of green silk cloth over the abdomen for one minute and then a piece of red silk cloth for one minute for a total of ten minutes (while lying in full sunlight); or lie in the Sun under a glass sheet of the appropriate color; or lie in the Sun with a lamp shining on the body using the appropriately colored bulb. I have found placing a silk cloth of the appropriate color on my body while lying in the Sun to be the most convenient of these methods.

3. **Food:** Fast lightly, eating only **Carrot juice** and **Melons** for seven days. You may also drink water and herb teas and take vitamins while fasting.

4. **Water:** For color treatments using water, Sun-solarize two quarts of water, using the colors yellow and green. You can either wrap one bottle of water in a piece of yellow silk and the other in green, or you can use yellow and green bottles. The bottles should be in the Sun for at least two weeks. Twice a day after drinking your juice, drink two ounces of the yellow-solarized water. When the tumor starts to recede, use the green water.

5. **Sleep:** You can use green cotton sheets for sleeping to enhance the Colortherapy and wear (mainly) green clothes.

The Special Get-Rid-of-Your-Problem-Within-One-Week Therapy

(According to exotic sources that have had results.)

Begin on a Monday, end on a waning moon Monday.

1. **Oil**—Sun-solarize two quarts of pure virgin **Olive oil,** one in red glass and one in green glass. Ideally they have been in the Sun for at least forty days but even three days will help.

Mix the two oils together and rub the tumor or abdominal area several times per day. Rub vigorously. (I would also add DMSO [dimethyl sulfoxide] to the oils: 8 oz mixed oil, 2 oz DMSO, ½ oz **Rose Geranium oil.**)

2. **Aromatherapy**—Put **Rose Geranium oil** in the vaporizer every night for sleeping.

3. **Color sleep**—Use pure cotton flannel green sheets for sleeping, preferably in green color (not lemon-green or blue-green).

4. **Air**—Alternate red and green air color baths for ten minutes once a day. Use red for one minute and then green for one minute. (If using silk cloths to cover the body when in the Sun, scent the red silk with herbs or essential oils of **Rose, Geranium,** or **Jasmine** and scent the green with **Narcissus, Galbanum,** or **Citronella.**)

5. **Gemstones**—Wear color-scented red/Topaz and green/ Emerald. Make sure the stones are in contact with the body directly.

6. **Diet**—Go on a one-week fast of **Carrot juice** and **Melons.** Eat and drink only these two items. You may take as much of each as you like. **Carrot juice** should be freshly pressed and drunk four to five times per day.

7. **Water**—Sun-solarize two quarts of water, one under yellow light and one under green light. Set in the Sun three to seven days. Drink 2 oz of yellow water after the juice or **Melon** twice a day during the acute phase. When the tumor starts to recede, switch to green water.

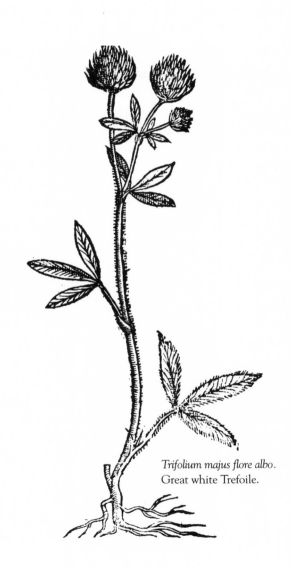

Trifolium majus flore albo.
Great white Trefoile.

Chapter 8

Pregnancy and Childbirth

The **Guelder Rose** is used as a uterine sedative,[19] especially when a miscarriage is threatening and for dysmenorrhea. This plant is particularly interesting to herbalists because it has been closely studied. The folk remedy of using the crude bark as tea has been shown to be stronger and more effective than the powdered extract prepared under laboratory conditions.[19] This is extremely interesting because herbalists feel that an entire plant must be used, rather than any one of its "active" components. Inherent factors in the natural plant, usually unknown or undiscovered, act in conjunction with each other in affecting the human body. In this particular plant the ancient herbal knowledge has proven true.

Raspberry leaf contains fragarine, a uterine relaxant, and is the standard herb used as a tea throughout pregnancy and lactation.

For morning sickness, use antispasmodic herbs such as **Peppermint, Catnip,** and **Chamomile** as teas. **Hops,** which has been thought to contain estrogens,[21] usually does not.[20] It provides a soothing antispasmodic action as a tea, as do **Basil herb** and **Raspberry leaf.**

Some herbs having strong medicinal qualities that may harm the developing fetus are best avoided during pregnancy, but can be used with knowledgeable guidance. **Pennyroyal, Tansy, Black**

Cohosh, Blue Cohosh, Yarrow, Mistletoe, Wild Celery, Rue, Peyote, Squaw Vine, and **Uva Ursi** are examples.

Some of the herbs that can be used during pregnancy include: **Alfalfa** and **Clover,** both of which contain phytoestrogens,[8] **Nettle** (iron in an easily assimilable form) for its nutritive value,[22] **Plantain** for potash, **Raspberry leaf** to tone the uterine muscle, and **Peach leaf** for nausea.

At birthing time many midwives use **Basil, Lavender,** and **Nutmeg** as a tea.[23] **Evening Primrose oil** applied to the cervix softens it and primes it for expansion. Drinking **Basil** tea helps expel the placenta. After the birth, drinking herb teas of **Comfrey leaf, Fennel seed, Nettle tops,** and **Alfalfa herb** encourages milk production.

If the baby has runny eyes, use a mixture of **Comfrey root*** and **Fennel seed** as an eyewash. Carefully strain the infusion to ensure that all herbal bits and pieces are removed from the liquid (tea).

For mastitis a hot poultice of **Comfrey root, Mullein flowers**, or **Lobelia** works very well. **Comfrey root,** especially if freshly grated, is preferable. Apply the warm poultice until the breast is red. Occasionally, if the breast is very sore you can apply the **Comfrey** poultice ice-cold to relieve the swelling.

For plentiful breast milk, a California midwife married to an obstetrician recommends the herbs **Marshmallow root** to strengthen the milk, **Blessed Thistle** to increase the flow, and **Nettle tops** and **Comfrey leaf**[5] to build up the blood. Europeans use **Fennel seed** and **Anise seed** to improve the flow of breast milk.

---

*For **Comfrey leaf** use only *Symphytum officinalis.* Other species can be harmful to the liver.

Aromatherapy Treatments for Pregnancy and Childbirth

Pregnancy and Nausea

Nausea due to pregnancy can be combatted by eating five small meals rather than three big ones, drinking **Chamomile** and **Red Raspberry leaf** tea at night before bed so that you won't be nauseous in the morning, and inhaling the essential oils of **Chamomile** and **Lavender** via a diffusor or simply from a handkerchief. The handkerchief must be kept in a plastic bag or the essential oils, which are volatile, will evaporate.

Your Stretching Belly and Breasts

The skin of the belly and the breasts should be rubbed every single day with **Coconut oil** that has vitamin E added to it or **Calendula**-infused oil* with the essential oils of **Mandarin, Tangerine,** or **Jasmine** added. Two drops of the essential oil per ounce of carrier oil is sufficient for a treatment. This will minimize stretch marks and toughen the breasts for the nursing process.

Labor

Labor can be eased by inhalation of various oils to suit the mood and time during the birthing process. Some midwives suggest inhaling the oils of **Basil** and **Lavender** for stimulation and relaxation, respectively. When the labor process is slowed by tension, whether muscular or nervous, take **Celery seed oil,** seven drops in a glass of water. Sip this between contractions.

---

*Directions for making **Calendula**-infused oil can be found in *The Aromatherapy Book: Applications & Inhalations* by Jeanne Rose. See information on Aromatherapy and Herbal Studies Course/Herbal Studies Library, in Source List, p. 121.

Perineal Tear

This can be minimized by dripping Olive oil on the perineum. Don't touch it, just take an eyedropper filled with Olive oil and drip one drop at a time on the perineal area as the baby begins to stretch this area. This will keep the tissue moist and elastic.

Can You Determine the Gender of Your Baby?

Some midwives argue that a determined-to-be-pregnant woman can indeed determine the gender of the baby. Since I have never tried these methods personally, I can only report what has been said to me.

A female baby is determined by an acid environment and a male baby by an alkaline environment. For a female child, have sexual intercourse two days before ovulation and precede this with a vinegar and water douche. For a male baby, increase the vaginal secretions with a mild baking soda douche. This seems to encourage the sperm because of the alkalinity of the vagina after the douching and by making the secretions more alkaline. Also have intercourse at ovulation itself.

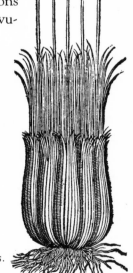

For more herbal child care, read the appropriate chapter in *Jeanne Rose's Modern Herbal*.

Nardus Narbonenfis.
French Spikenard.

Chapter 9

Seven Steps to Healing Cysts, Vague Aches, Menorrhagia

Several years ago after a particularly emotional time in my life when my mother had died, my boyfriend had died, I was getting a divorce, and my children were not particularly interesting or nice (in fact, acting like children), my health deteriorated. My menstrual cycle became very erratic. My breasts ached and oozed a milky fluid and developed lumps. The OB/Gyn diagnosed fibrocystic disease of the uterus as well as the breast and sent me to a surgeon because my breasts were "suspicious." The surgeon, looking worried, asked me to come in every two weeks to palpate my breasts. He discussed all the options regarding breast surgery—cysts that might be cancerous or not, breasts that might be cut off or left on, etc. These are terrifying words to any woman. I immediately went off in five different directions to investigate all the current medical as well as alternative treatments.

I determined that my period (menstrual cycle) would have to be stabilized and that the cause of its erratic behavior was fluctuating hormones. (This was, of course, not "scientific" fact, but who cares when what you do determines whether or not you will keep or have your breasts or uterus cut off or out.) With herbs and vitamin supplements I stabilized my period and reduced the cysts on both my uterus and breasts. Massage increased the value of the herbs, and for good measure, I underwent a series of acupuncture treatments and also took the advice of a homeo-path. The entire course of this treatment took a year, but after-ward the surgeon declared that the cysts on my breasts were "almost nonexistent," my menstrual cycle had stabilized at a very regular twenty-six days with the day of ovulation always occurring on the evening of the twelfth day, there was no longer any pain or swelling in my breasts during the progesterone phase of the cycle, and no "breakthrough" bleeding (bleeding that occurs during the middle of the cycle). These measures worked for me and would work for most women if used *consistently* over a period of time. They should be tried by any woman who faces the loss of any of her reproductive organs.

1. **Diet**—Change the diet to one that is mostly vegetarian, comprised of 70–80% alkaline-forming foods. Eat grains for breakfast, a large meal at noon that includes protein (deep-water ocean fish, Almonds, or chicken), and primarily vegetables at dinner (salad, a steamed vegetable, and a baked Potato). Fruits should be kept for snacks and an Apple consumed every morn-ing about an hour before breakfast. Delete from the diet all stim-ulants like caffeine drinks (cola, Coffee, Black Tea, Chocolate) and drugs such as nicotine and alcohol. Remember that some researchers state unequivocally that breast cysts are caused by rancid fats in the diet. Rancid fats, which most Americans seem to eat in abundance, also cause colon cancer.

2. **Vitamin Supplements**—Take anti-oxidants every day to reduce the risk and counteract rancid fats. Include 1–10 grams per day of vitamin C, 400–800 units of D-Alpha tocopherol (vitamin E), 150 mg of Selenium, brewer's yeast, bone meal (at least 1200 mg of calcium), 25–100 mg each of zinc derived from zinc gluconate, and a good supplement that includes all other vitamins and minerals, especially B_6. Often estrogen is not being metabolized properly in women with erratic menstrual cycles and/or breast lumps, and these women must be regulated with diet and supplements. Take 50 mg of B_6 daily to aid in the metab-

olization of estrogen, increasing the dosage during the latter part of the cycle. I found that I could immediately reduce the aching in my breasts by taking a 50-mg B_6 tablet. I often took up to 300 mg of B_6 after ovulation. Generally, time-release tablets of vitamin C and B_6 work more efficiently than those that dissolve quickly. Take bioflavinoids and Kelp along with the vitamin C.

3. **Exercise**—Exercise, and do it every day. The more you exercise the better you will feel.

4. **Herbs**—Drink the Estrogen Stimulating Tea and Progesterone Stimulating Tea on page 28. Use the Estrogen Tea only if necessary. Take the Progesterone Tea in increasing doses from a few days before ovulation until menstruation begins. Take one cup per day prior to ovulation, then two cups a day during ovulation, three cups a day until the day of menstruation, and then stop. Another Progesterone Tea formula that worked well for me was a mixture of the following:

> 4 oz each of **Raspberry leaf** and **Sarsaparilla root**
> 2 oz each of **Rosemary leaf, Holy Thistle tops,** and
>   **Nettle tops**
> 1 oz each of **Ginseng root** and **Sandalwood bark**

This total of 16 oz should last the user two months. Use ½ oz herbs per quart of water per day.

Using the Chinese system of influencing the organs, take the tea in the afternoon between the hours of 3:00 P.M. and 5:00 P.M. I alternated this formulation with another progesterone-stimulating herb tea that included the following:

> 4 oz each of **Sarsaparilla** and **Aralia (Spikenard)**
> 2 oz each of **Raspberry, Rosemary,** and **Nettle**
> 1 oz each of **Oatstraw** and **Ginseng**

½ oz herbs per quart of water in a standard infusion. Drink 1 quart of tea per day.

Frankly, I cannot tell which of these three formulations worked most effectively.

Another important herb and animal supplement for any woman over the age of thirty is raw female tissue, a glandular supplement. This can be purchased in any health food store and usually contains a mixture of herbal supplements along with ovarian and uterine tissue. Take three tablets per week.

Use the Basic Bolus Formula for at least six months to draw out acid wastes in the uterus and to reduce cysts. Use the Basic YEGG Formula for ten days out of every month for at least six months.

5. **Color**—Use the color cure already outlined once every three months.

6. **Aromatherapy**—If you have cancer, use a vaporizer every night while you sleep and put **Rose Geranium oil** or **Thuja oil***
in the well. A few drops will do. **Clary Sage oil** is also useful. These are soothing to the psyche and will help you sleep.

7. **Massage**—Vigorous massage helps to dissipate the cysts, whether in the breast or the uterus. Every night rub your breasts vigorously in a circular motion with Olive oil mixed with a lit-tle **Rose Geranium oil.** Or you can use the color-treated oil mentioned in Step 1, Chapter 7, and add the **Rose Geranium** essential oil to it. (Another treatment I have used is B_6 mashed to a paste in a bit of DMSO (to facilitate passage). Rub this on the breast vigorously for three to five minutes three times per day.)

---

*__Thuja oil__ is considered toxic and should *only* be used in a very serious situation or not at all.

Chapter 10

Menopause

The menopause is the time in a woman's life when her child-bearing years are over. This usually occurs in the early fifties although there are many women who begin menopause in their forties. Menstruation ceases and with that a whole host of hormonal changes occur in the woman. Menopause is also called the climacteric, and though I well know that climacteric relates to the word climax or end—that is, the end of childbearing years (notwithstanding the fact that physicians around the world are artificially creating childbearing women in their sixties)—I continue to think that climacteric really has to do with the inner *climate* of the menopausal woman.

Many women experience this change in their life with little to no discomfort. The inner climate just slowly changes, adjusting easily to the new hormonal surges and lack of surges. Some women, however, experience many changes and health problems related to the drop in estrogen and progesterone levels. These symptoms include those famous hot flashes, depression, palpitations of the heart, joint pain, foot pain, fattening of the abdominal and thigh area, night sweats, bone loss resulting in osteoporosis, cold chills, and all sorts of other symptoms. In addition, the secretions in the vagina dry up often causing painful sexual intercourse.

How can we get through menopause and this change in our inner climate with little or no effort? I think that the answer lies in the litany of good health: take regular exercise, eat a balanced whole-food diet, drink clean water, breathe pure air, lead a full life, and be *satisfied* with your condition.

If you do have some of the problems of menopause that no amount of exercise, food, vitamins, and smiles will heal, here are some of the remedies.

Hot Flashes

The problem with women who complain about hot flashes is that they do not understand that a "hot flash" is an out-of-body experience. They are actually quite exciting, and I think of them, when I am fortunate enough to have one, as "psychedelic rivulets of heat."* Warmth and heat flow over the entire body. My mom never told me that a "hot flash" could be "hot and flashing." I guess our parents did not have experience with psychedelics.

Maybe we get these psychedelic rivulets of heat bouncing off our heads and ears because the "inner" climate no longer can adjust the thermostat of the body. The hypothalamus just doesn't know when to adjust. The remedies for this situation include spritzing your face and ears with the hydrosols of Peppermint, Lemon Verbena, or Rose Geranium. Do this immediately as you feel the hot flash coming on. If you do not have hydrosols handy, simply add 2 drops of Peppermint oil to 4 ounces of pure distilled water, shake, refrigerate, and use this to spritz your burning cheeks and sweating body whenever necessary. Shirley Price in her wonderful *Aromatherapy Workbook* also suggests "Hot Flash Water." This is one quart of spring water to which you have added 4 drops of essential oil of Peppermint. Shake care-

---

*[**Editor's Note:** This was written in 1986 just as Jeanne began taking the anti-inflammatory drug Prednisone to control a dangerous condition in her lungs, and now she gets hot and bothered, and the rest of us have to endure air conditioning and wide open windows in the dead of winter!!]

fully, keep cool. Whenever you feel a hot flash coming on quickly drink 4 ounces of the water and splash a bit on your face.

Inhale **Clary Sage oil** and alternate this with **Grapefruit oil.**

Balance the Hormonal Output

Make a decoction of 1 part of each of the following herbs: **False Unicorn root, Ginseng root, Black Cohosh, Blue Cohosh, *Vitex Agnus Castus* seeds, Blessed Thistle, Wild Yam,** and ½ part of **Licorice.** Drink 2 cups of this daily.

Dry Vagina

This condition can be eased by applying egg white prior to intercourse or a vitamin E oil mixed with **Comfrey root** ointment. **Rose oil** can be added to vitamin E oil and applied to the labia as an alternate remedy.

Relieving Emotional States Using Aromatherapy*

The Olfactory Research Fund announced results of a study showing that daily use of scent can help the five common mood states of menopause: tension-anxiety, depression-dejection, anger-hostility, fatigue-inertia, and confusion-bewilderment. Essential oils can be inhaled or applied externally. The use of scent "opens up" the sensory systems and "allows positive emotions to flow."

Ylang-Ylang oil can be inhaled as an antidepressant or sleep-inducer. Applied to a handkerchief and inhaled, it reduces tension, anxiety, depression, and anger, and can stimulate adrenal glands. It acts as an aphrodisiac and stimulant to the immune system, calms nerves, is euphoric and sedative, soothes anger, reduces physical pain, and is used to treat insomnia. **Ylang-Ylang oil** can be used externally in lotions, massage oils, and baths as a relaxant and is soothing to jangled nerves. One drop of **Ylang-**

---

*These oils are contained in Jeanne Rose's Aromatherapy First-Aid Kit™ for Women's Care. See Source List, p. 123.

Ylang oil in honey daily is taken internally as a treatment for impotence and frigidity.

Geranium oil is inhaled to stimulate the adrenal cortex, to reduce symptoms of asthma and menopause, and to stimulate the thyroid for weight loss. **Geranium** treats depression, dejection, fatigue, inertia, confusion and bewilderment, and all anxiety states, balances adrenals, balances hormones, has a harmonious effect, calms and refreshes, and uplifts the body and psyche. Externally **Geranium oil** is used in facial steams, lotions, massage oils, and baths to treat the face and body, especially dry to normal and normal to oily skin. It balances all functions of the oil glands. **Geranium oil** is healing and antiseptic. It is used for massage to ease PMS or cramps. It is an excellent all-purpose essential oil for the skin of women young and old, as well as children.

Chamomile and **Lavender oil** can be mixed and is the prime all-purpose women's oil. It is inhaled to soothe and calm, to ease depression, and to soothe irritability. One drop on the forehead is relaxing and allays bad temper. It is soothing to children. **Chamomile** and **Lavender oil** is calming, used for headache and migraines, works as a stress reducer and relaxing agent, and leaves peaceful feelings. Externally **Chamomile** and **Lavender oil** has many skin uses including soothing inflammation. It is used in facial steams to cleanse the pores and calm acne, in baths and washes to reduce puffiness, in massage oils to reduce muscular aches and pain. It eases pain in the reproductive system and anywhere in the body.

Clary Sage oil is inhaled as an adrenal stimulant. It eases depression, reduces hot flashes, helps the new mother relax, and is mildly intoxicating. With **Geranium oil,** it is good for menopause symptoms, eases nervousness, and soothes PMS symptoms. It is relaxing and euphoric, and with **Ylang-Ylang** is used for menstrual irregularities, for reducing wrinkles, and applied to hair roots to stimulate growth. **Clary Sage** is used in the bath for health and relaxation. Dilute with water and spritz on the face for hot skin and during heat waves. As a massage it encourages the labor process and strengthens the kidneys and stomach. It is very good for all menstrual disorders. Internally one drop in warm water is a gargle for sore throat. When you get tired of **Clary Sage oil** alternate with **Grapefruit oil.**

Aching Feet

There is one other symptom of menopause that I have never seen mentioned, and that is aching feet, heel spurs, and pain across the top of the arch. These pains can be so bad that women can't walk easily. I feel certain that these problems relate to the hormonal changes that are occurring as well as to bone loss or lack of calcium in the diet. I have devised several methods to combat this problem including the addition of calcium, magnesium, vitamin E, and B_6, which we have already discussed.

Herbal treatments include massage rubs with products that contain the herbs and essential oils of **Rosemary, Comfrey,** and other treatments of this type. This is very helpful.

My favorite method incorporates the use of essential oils in a foot soak followed by a rub of **Lavender oil.** Personally, I use the Herbal Hydrotherapy Foot Revival Soak made by ABRA Baths in Guerneville, CA. This really should be called Aromatherapy Treatment for Feet, as it is so effective. Call (707) 869-0761 to find your nearest outlet for this product.

Foot Revival Soak contains a therapeutic quantity of herbal extracts of **Arnica flowers, White Willow bark,** and **Lemon Balm leaves** and therapeutic quantities of essential oils of **Peppermint, Sage, Eucalyptus, Clove buds,** and **Balsam of Peru** in a bath salt base. Soak your feet every evening in this solution, dry them, rub them with true **Lavender** oil, and put on a pair of socks. This is a fabulous treatment that in time will heal those aching feet.

Women's Health vs. Horses
Estrogen Boom Brings Breeding Horses for Slaughter

Adapted from *Animal People*, 1993.

Rocketing demand for estrogen replacement drugs is expected to double the number of farms producing pregnant mare's urine (PMU) from 300 in 1991 to 7000 by the end of 1994. Already, almost 500 farms are collecting urine from an estimated 75,000 catheterized mares. Because the mares must be pregnant to produce a commercially viable amount of estrogen, they will give birth to as many as 90,000 foals this year—most of them in April, since the equine gestation cycle normally runs from September to April.

Most of these foals will be sold for meat. The foals are sold at four to five months of age and trucked long distances for slaughter. At that time the mothers are re-impregnated. Fillies who show temperament and conformation to become PMU producers are kept as replacements for worn out or infertile mares or are used to expand production.

The estrogen is used in PMU-based estrogen replacement drugs. Estrogen is collected from the PMU and then concentrated and shipped to a manufacturing plant. The business emerged in the 1960s when birth control pills went into widespread use, and is booming again because PMU is the base material of the synthetic hormonal drug, Premarin, prescribed to menopausal women. As the Baby Boomers who supported the birth control industry reach middle age, Premarine therapy is expected to become one of the most lucrative drug markets.

Critics of PMU manufacturing state that the investment only adds 71 industrial jobs to the economy, the waste overburdens the sewage system, the industry is cruel to animals, and the promotion of Premarin in itself may involve risks to women's health, as birth control pills were found to have harmful side effects for many women after prolonged use. The critics cite the link between estrogen replacement therapy (ERT) and endometrial cancer. Women's health experts now recommend that Premarin be prescribed only to deal with osteoporosis and other serious medical conditions, not simply to ease normal menopause. The preferred approach to these as well as normal conditions of menopause is preventive diet and exercise.

The living conditions of the mares are similar to those of intensively raised dairy cattle. The mares are confined to their stalls for more than half of each year, and can only stand up and sit down for exercise. Sanitary conditions are monitored, mostly for public image reasons, so that horse abuse scandal, similar to those which killed the PMU industry 23 years ago, can be avoided.

Horse expert Sharon Cragier states that the code of ethics for sanitary conditions are insufficient to guarantee PMU-producing horses even the minimal comfort possible when spending six-plus months tethered, catheterized, and pregnant. She believes the recommended stall size is a foot too narrow to allow the average mare to enjoy deep sleep, while the recommended brush concrete flooring may cause sore hooves.

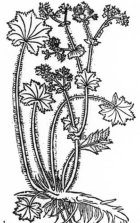

Alchimilla.
Lyons-foot, or Ladies Mantle.

Simple Formulas During Menopause

Formula #1

> Equal quantities of **Licorice root, Angelica (Don Quai*) root, Black Cohosh root, Sarsaparilla root, Ginseng root, Blessed Thistle tops, False Unicorn root,** and **Spikenard root.**

Formula #2

> One part each of **Wild Yam root, False Unicorn root, Licorice root, Comfrey root, True Unicorn root, Life Root or False Valerian, Angelica root,** and **Rosemary leaf.**
>
> ½ part each of **Spikenard,**[24] **Sarsaparilla, Blessed Thistle tops, Ginseng,** and **Red Clover.**

Mix the dried herbs together, bottle in a light-proof container, label, and store in a dark, cool place. The general dosage is one cup of tea twice a day. Make the tea in the usual way— 1 T of the mixed herbs simmered in 1 cup of water for 1 minute and then removed from the heat, cooled to room temperature, strained, and drunk. Add honey, if you like. Use the residue of herbs for the second cup of tea. It is also important to take B_6 and bone meal and to get PLENTY of exercise.

This time in a woman's life can be a particularly difficult time. Often simply increasing the vitamin supplements that ease stress may be all that is necessary for relief. B_6 seems to be especially helpful. The mixtures of herbs used in treating menopause are various combinations of plants that provide phytoestrogens

---

*Don Quai is spelled in a variety of ways, including Dong Quai.

and progesterone precursors. The estrogenic herbs predominate. Use whichever tea works best.

Don't forget to exercise and eat properly, taking at least 2000 mg of calcium and 600 mg of magnesium every night before bedtime, plus zinc, B_6, and vitamin C.

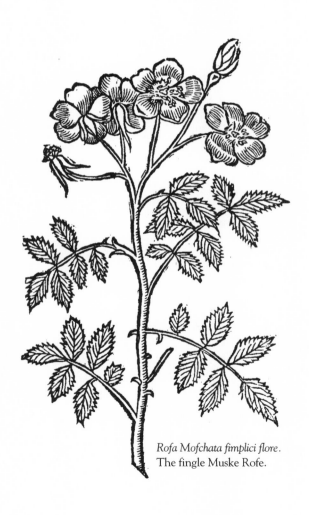

Rofa Mofchata fimplici flore.
The fingle Muske Rofe.

Notes

Notes to Text

1. *Webster's Third New International Dictionary*, Philip Go, Editor-in-Chief. (Springfield, Mass: C&G Merriam & Co., 1965). (used for all definitions)

2. "Naturally-Occurring Estrogens in Plant Foodstuffs, A Review," Kathey Verdeal and Dales Ryan, *Journal of Food Protection*, Vol. 42, No. 7 (July, 1979): 577–583.

3. "Premenstrual water retention. Favorable effect of Agnus castus (Agnolyt) on premenstrual water retention." *Index Medicus* 55 (1), 48–51, (1979) 10.

4. "Acne vulgaris and Agnus castus." *Index Medicus* 51 (35), 1645–8, (Dec. 1975) 20.

5. "Pharmacological investigation of the essential oil of *Daucus carota* var. *sativa*," A. K. Bhargava, S. M. Ali, and C. S. Chauhan (Univ. Saugar, Sagar), *Indian J. Pharm.* 29 (4), (1967): 127–9.

6. "Naturally Occurring Estrogens in Plant Foodstuffs, A Review," Kathey Verdeal and Dales Ryan. *Journal of Food Protection* 42, No. 7 (July, 1979): 577–583.

7. "Estrogenic activity of Glycyrrhiza glabra and Glycyrrhiza uralensis hay," Goryachev, V. S., Pauzner, L. E., Muinova, S. S. *Mater. Biol. Vidov Roda Glycyrrhiza L.*, (1970): 11–15.

8. "Estrogen activity of some fodder plants in northern Ossetia," Taskaev, A. Kh. (Gorskii S.-Kh. Inst., Ordzhonikidze, USSR). Rast. Resur. 1971, 7 (2): 295–8.

9. "Estrogenic properties of Glycyrrhiza glabra (licorice)," Murav'ev, I. A., Kononikhina, N. F. (Pyatigorsk, Farm. Inst.,m Pyatigorsk, USSR). Rast. Resur. 1972, 8 (4): 490–7.

10. "Effect of plant estrogens on the reproductive system of rabbits," Madoyan, O. O., Mkrtchyan, S. A., Markaryan, S. G., Prazyan, K. A., Bagdasarova, L. A. (Nauchno-Issled, Inst. Zhivotnovod. Vet., Erevan, USSR). *Izu Sel'skokhoz. Nauk*, 1973, 16 (2): 67–72.

11. "Review on chemical and medicinal aspects of *Allium sativum*," Ikram, M. (Pakistan Counc. Sci. Ind. Res. Lab., Peshawar, Pak.). *Pak. J. Sci. Ind. Res.*, 1972, 15 (1–2): 81–6.

12. "Effect of garlic in the diet on the intestinal microflora of rats," Subrahmanhan, V., Krishnamurthy, K., Sree-Nivasamurthy, V., and Swaminathan, M. *J. Sci. Indust. Res.*, 1957, 16C: 173–174.

13. "Antimicrobial properties of garlic," Kabelik, Jan (Reg. Admin. Public Health, Centre Hyg. Epidemiol., Olemouc, Czech.), *Pharmazie*, 1970, 25 (4): 266–70.

14. "Data on the fungicidal and fungistatic action in vitro phytocides of onion and garlic on geotrichoid," Lesnikov, E. P. *Byull. Ekspll. Biol. Med.*, 24 (1), 70–2 (1947).

15. "Comparative determination of arbutoside in some species from the family Ericaceae from Stara Planina." Mihajlov, M., Janackovic-Milojevic, B. (Inst. Res. Med. Plants, Belgrade, Yugoslavia), *Lek. Sirovine*, 1968, 6: 57–64.

16. "Studies on Vaccinium myrtinus anthocyanosides II. Aspects of anthocyanins pharmacokinetics in the rat." Lietti, A., Forni, G. (Res. Lab., Inverni Beffa, Milan, Italy). *Arzneim-Forsch.*, 1976, 26 (5): 832–5.

17. *Guide to Medicinal Plants.* Schauenberg and Paris. (Keats Publishing, Inc., New Canaan, Conn.: (Original French edition, 1974.) 1977).

18. "Anthocyanin glucosides." Laboratories Chibret. Belg. 615–972, July 30, 1962; Fr. Appl. Apr. 18, 1961: 13.

19. "Viburnum Studies. XVI. Rate of extraction of uterine sedative potency," Sloane, Aaron B., Latven, Albert R., and Munch, James C. *J. Am. Pharm. Assoc.* 38, (1949).

20. "Is estrogenic activity present in hops?" Fenselau, Catherine, Talalay, P., Sch. Med., Johns Hopkins Univ., Baltimore, Md.). *Food Cosmet. Toxicol.* 1973, 11 (4), 597–603.

21. "Estrogenic hops extract for cosmetics." Strenkovskaya, A.G. (Moscow Scientific-Research Institute of Cosmetology), USSR 219, 112 (Cl. A 61K), 30 May 1968, Appl. 28 Apr. 1967; from *Izobret., Prom, Obrazlsy, Toyarnyc Znaki*, 1968, 45 (18), 57.

22. "Chemical composition and nutritive value of leafy vegetables underutilized in Bulgaria." Obretenova, N., Kepova, D., Petrova, K., Kolev, N., Kurdzhieva, N. (Inst. Khranene, Sofia, Bulg.) *Izv. Inst., Khranene, Bulg. Akad. Nauk.* (1973) 11, 5–20.

23. Handouts for Natural Childbirth Preparation. Koehler, Solomon or Hunt. 13140 Frati Lane, Sebastopol, CA 95474.

24. "Natural groups of trace elements in medicinal plants having a tonic effect." Grinkevich, N. I., Koval'skii, V. V., Gribovskaya, I. F. (USSR).

Serdechno-Sosudistaya Patol. Bolez, Obmena Veshchestu, 1971: 168–78.

25. "Aristolochia," Horrisberger, P. (Biel, Switz.). *Schweiz. Apoth.-Zig.* 1971, 109 (11), 380–2.

26. "Pharmacological studies on herb Peony root. IV. Analysis of therapeutic effects of Peony and Licorice-containing common prescriptions in Chinese medicine and comparison with effects of experimental pharmacological tests." Harada, Masatoshi (Fac. Pharm. Sci., Univ. Chiba, Japan) *Yakugaku Zasshi* 1969, 89 (7) 899–908.

Additional References

"Antineoplastic agent from *Cnicus benedictus.*" Cobb, Edith M. Brit. 1, 335, 181 (Cl. A61k) 24 Oct. 1973, Appl, 54, 800/69, 08 Nov. 1969.

"Viopudial, a hypotensive and smooth muscle antispasmodic from *Viburnum opulus.*" Nicholson, John A., Darby, Thomas D., Jarboe, Charles H. (Sch. Med. Univ. Louisville, Louisville, KY). *Proc. Soc. Exp. Biol. Med.* 1972, 140 (2), 457–61.

"Beta-Radioactivity of the mineral constituents of medicinal herbs," Tadeusz Pelczat (Akad. Med., Cracow). Acta Polon, Pharm., 23 (2), 129–33 (1966).

"Enzymic extraction of anthocyanin glycosides," Pourrat, Henri, Pourrat, Aimee, Lamaison, J. L., Perrin, B. (Fac. Pharm., Clermont-Ferrand, Fr.). *Bull. Liaison, Groupe Polyphenols* (1973): 4.

"Estrogenicity in plants," Aharaf, A. (Pharmacol. Res. Unit, Nat. Res. Centre, UAR). *Arab Sci. Congr., 5th, Bagdad,* 1966 (Pub. 1967): (Pt. 1), 281–90.

"Estrogen effect of licorice root." Van Hulle, C. (Pharm. Inst., Reichsuniv. Cent. Ghent, Belg.). *Pharmazie* 1970, 25 (10), 260–1.

"Pharmacology of licorice root," Watanabe, Kazuo (Fac. Pharm. Sci., Toyama Univ., Toyama, Japan). *Taisha,* 10 (1973): 626–311.

"Estrogenic activity of fermented alfalfa," Jorgensen, N. A., Freymiller, D. D. (Dep. Dairy Sci., Univ. Wisconsin, Madison, WIS). *J. Dairy Sci.* 1972, 55 (1), 80–2.

"Interactions between phyto-estrogens and steroids in the cervical mucus and uterine eright responses in ewes" Kelly, R. W., Allison, A. J., Shirley, D. K. (Invermay Agric. Res. Cent., Minist. Agric. Fish., Mosgiel, N. Z.). *Aust. J. Agric. Res.,* 1976, 27 (1), 101–7.

Notes

Part II

THE MALE

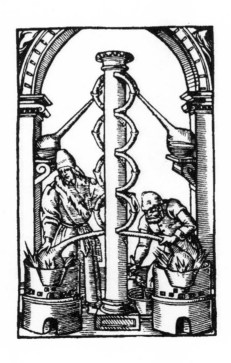

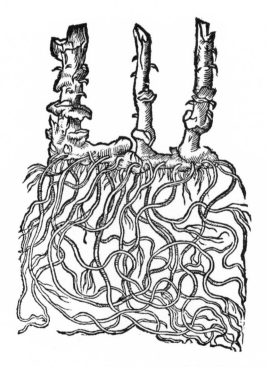

Smilax Peruviana, Salfaparilla.
Rough Binde-weed of Peru.

Chapter 11

Male Basics

Most of the male reproductive anatomy is external. The two testes hang in a sac called the scrotum. The testes have two functions, one of which is the production of sex hormones. Testosterone is the hormone which causes development of male sexual characteristics, and a little estrogen exists as a hormonal balance for the testosterone and for the production of spermatozoa.

The function of the testes is hindered by high temperature, which might be caused by shorts or jeans that are too tight. The normal temperature is lower than the abdominal cavity. Because the testes hang outside the body the temperature is regulated more easily.

About 200 million sperm are produced every day in the testes, then collected in the ducts which lead to the epididymis. In the epididymis the sperm spend about ten days maturing and then move to the *vas deferens* where they can live, if necessary, for another six weeks before degenerating and being absorbed.

Upon ejaculation, a variable number of sperm shoot through the *vas deferens* and pass through the seminal vesicles where various secretions are added, including those from the prostate gland. These secretions are rather alkaline in nature, somewhat neutralizing the acidity of the male urethra (from urine), as well as the normal acidity of the female vagina.

The prostate gland is one of two storage areas of zinc in the

73

body—the other being the retina of the eye. Zinc is a mineral that helps in the thinking process and aids in deodorizing sweat glands. Thus, "Zinc makes you think," and "Zinc keeps you from stinking."

The prostate lies at the base of the bladder. Other glands that produce a major part of the ejaculate are called Cowper's gland and Littre's gland. The ejaculate moves down the urethra through the penis where, if non-oral heterosexual unprotected intercourse is taking place, it can be deposited high in the vagina.

The penis is made up of the root, body, and the glans. It is composed of erectile tissue supplied with blood vessels. During sexual excitement the blood vessels in the erectile tissue become engorged with blood and the normally soft and limp penis becomes firm, sometimes hard, enlarging and expanding by about a third.

The glans is rich in nerve endings and thus very sensitive. In the circumcised male, the frenum, a nerve-packed gland, is removed as well as the foreskin. This reduces sexual sensitivity in the male as well as removes many lubricating sebaceous glands.

During erection the veins, which normally drain the erectile tissue, become blocked. This constriction maintains the erection until orgasm where it subsides, the veins drain, and the penis again becomes soft and small.

Drugs, especially cocaine, alcohol, and even nicotine, inhibit the erection of a sexually excited man. Other drugs with this effect include prescriptive medications to control heart arrhythmia, blood pressure, and other medical conditions.

Semen contains a mixture of chemicals, minerals, fructose, and various proteins which help with the nutrition of the sperm while in the vagina. The fructose in the semen is regulated by testosterone and seems to be essential to the movement of the sperm.

Chapter 12

Birth Control

A man can practice absolute birth control by having a vasectomy. In this procedure, the *vas deferens* are surgically cut, which blocks the passage of the spermatozoa but does not stop their production. Sperm build up, however, in the *vas deferens* where they inevitably have to degenerate and be absorbed. Recently evidence has been cropping up that vasectomy has other more serious health effects than simply sterilization. Studies done on monkeys fed a high-fat diet similar to that eaten by most American men show an association between vasectomy and arteriosclerosis (hardening of the arteries). Arteriosclerosis was even more severe in vasectomized monkeys fed a low-fat, no-cholesterol diet such as that eaten by men in third-world countries. Apparently the body forms antibodies against its own sperm, treating sperm like foreign bodies. The antibodies bind with the sperm or sperm fragments to eliminate them. The sperm or fragments are then deposited in the blood vessel, and this injures the vessel walls and begins the process leading to hardening.

Another way for a man to take part in the responsibility of conception, however, is to become intimately familiar with the body of the woman he is involved with. Men can learn to determine when a woman ovulates by seeing, feeling, touching, and tasting the changes that occur vaginally and cervically. The chart reflecting female hormonal phases in Chapter 2 should be studied. Thoughtful, loving, responsible men can also learn as easily as women how to put a diaphragm or cervical cap in place and to determine the time of ovulation.

The only other way in which a man can practice natural birth control is to become either celibate or homosexual.

How Not to Get Women Pregnant*

Male Sterilization (Vasectomy)

What: Tubes that deliver sperm are cut or blocked. **How:** Prevents sperm from traveling from testicles to penis. **Effectiveness:** 99%. **Satisfaction:** 90% general. **Plus:** none. **Minus:** Postsurgical pain and swelling; risk of infection (rare); does not protect against sexually transmitted diseases. **Caution:** Procedure is reversible; though it can fail to prevent pregnancy (very rare), vasectomy is generally more effective and less risky than female sterilization. **Minor surgery:** $250–550.

Future Contraceptives For Men

- Two **implants** in the upper arm, each good for a year and each releasing a different chemical; a peptide analog to suppress sperm production and diminish sex drive, and a chemical to maintain libido. Currently in FDA-approved clinical trials.

- A **vaccine** that would suppress sperm production without diminishing sex drive via a series of injections. FDA-approved trials underway.

- New **polyurethane** or **Tactylon condoms** would address the needs of men and women who are allergic to latex, while offering equivalent protection against sexually transmitted diseases.

---

*By permission of Ruth Mayer, adapted from *Mademoiselle* Magazine, August 1993.

Chapter 13

Herbs for Males

There are not as many herbs listed in the literature and reper-
tory of herbalists for men as there are for women. Although a
woman's hormonal cycle is very complicated, men also produce
hormones that can be adversely affected by many different things.
The male hormone testosterone causes development of the characteristics that make a man a man—bulkier muscles, facial hair,
a deeper voice, and aggressiveness. The interstitial cells of the
testis also produce some of the female hormone, estrogen.

Herbs, drugs, medicines, foods—all can affect the male reproductive system. During the last few years I have counseled many
men on their inability to get an erection and have found that
usually one of two situations exists. The men may enjoy taking
recreational drugs and consider marijuana and cocaine to be
aphrodisiacal. However, too much of either of these substances
reduces sensitivity, causing a temporary inability to become
erect. In the case of cocaine this inability can last as long as six
hours after the last "line" has been snorted (inhaled). The other
simple reason is performance anxiety—too much sex, or too
much with too many in too short a time. The penis just gives
up for a while.

Herbs and moderation in lifestyle can help these and all sorts
of other problems.

Anemone pulsatilla, also called the **Pasque flower** or **Wind**

flower, is a general stimulant to the entire system. It encourages all the secretions of the body from spit to urine, and in women, encourages milk production and the menses as well. In men it is used to treat inflammation of the testis (orchitis) and inflammation of the prostate (prostatitis). It is quite a powerful medicine, and generally taken in tincture form, ten drops at a time in a bit of water, twice a day.

Bearberry *(Arctostaphylos uva-ursi),* an herb usually considered a specific for the kidney, has great value as a tea for the health of the prostate as well. It gives strength and tone to all the urinary passages.

Black Cohosh very strongly affects the central nervous system of both men and women. It is an important part of any formula treating an erection problem. **Black Willow** *(Salix nigra)* is often used with **Black Cohosh.** It acts as a sedative and tonic. **Boneset** *(Eupatorium purpureum)* is used with **Bearberry** when there is irritation in the urinary passages and especially when the prostate is enlarged or inflamed.

Burdock *(Arctium lappa)* is the herb of choice for all skin conditions. All parts are used—seed, herb, root, and flowers. The seed and leaf (herb) are used externally in powder form for scrotal eczema and taken internally for prostatitis and epididymitis. The seeds are mainly used for skin conditions such as sebaceous cysts, while the root is used for deeper conditions. The Chinese use the root to promote secretions, as an alternative treatment in syphilis, and externally on chronic sores. They use the seed tincture both internally and applied externally for long-standing skin conditions such as psoriasis.

Cornsilk (the stigmas from **red Indian corn,** *Zea mays*) is used with other herbs that affect the urinary passage. It, too, works well with **Uva-ursi** and **Boneset.** This combination—**Cornsilk, Uva-ursi, Boneset**—is an excellent formula for inflamed urinary passages in both men and women, affecting the prostate and other glands of reproductive secretions as well.

Damiana *(Turnera aphrodisiaca)* is a general stimulant and sexual tonic. In Mexico an alcoholic beverage called Crema de Damiana is made and sold as an aphrodisiac (tongue-in-cheek, of course, except to those men who buy it and drink it and find out that it is indeed very effective). **Damiana** works well with **Saw Palmetto** *(Serenoa repens)*. They are generally used together in equal parts. **Saw Palmetto berries** are used as a tonic and when combined with **Damiana** have a beneficial effect on the male reproductive organs; the combination seems to build strength and increase flesh.

Ginseng *(Panax schinseng)*, a root indigenous to the East, has been used for thousands of years as a medicine for the lymphatic and the reproductive system. In small doses it stimulates the nerve centers of the *medulla oblongata*, stimulates the sympathetic nervous system, increases metabolism, stimulates the smooth muscle fiber, increases erection ability, retards impotence, and regulates blood pressure and blood sugar as well as performing in many other ways in the human system. The usual dose is 5–10 grams in a decoction every morning before breakfast. **Black Tea** and iron supplements are considered incompatible with **Ginseng** therapy.

Groundsel *(Senecio vulgaris)*, a simple plant generally considered a noxious weed, is used for any problems with the male sexual organ.

In Brazil **Muira-puama** *(Liriosma ovata)* **root** is used as an aphrodisiac and nerve stimulant. It can be drunk as a tea and used with **Saw Palmetto, Damiana,** and **Ginseng.**

Myrtle *(Myrtus communis)* is generally considered a women's herb to increase secretions, but it can be used for this purpose as well by men when there is a diminution of sexual fluids.

Rhododendron, a common flower, has been used often in herbal medicine, although it is not much in favor now. It is one of the few plants that seems to be effective in treating a *hydrocele* (a collection of fluid other than blood or pus in the scrotum). Use a tea daily of **Rhododendron** and a combination of other herbs as a poultice externally.

Saw Palmetto Berries *(Serenoa repens* **or** *S. serrulata).*
The berry of this palm is used as a nutritive, diuretic, and urinary antiseptic. It especially affects the genito-urinary system
of men. James Green in *The Male Herbal* says that it "safely and
efficiently tones and strengthens the male reproductive system,
enhancing the male sex hormones." It is used specifically to
treat the prostate gland, especially when it is enlarged and debil-
itated. It increases bladder tone and allows a better contraction,
and thereby a more complete expulsion of bladder contents.
The dose is 1 cup of the infusion three times per day. If you prefer the tincture, use 25–30 drops 3x/day or take two of the size
00 capsules of the ground-up berries 3x/day.

Thuja occidentalis, also called **Arbor Vitae** or **Tree of Life,**
the herb is used as a blood tonic and if mixed with **Oats** *(Avena*
sativa) can stimulate the nerves. **Thuja** is used to treat many
chronic conditions of the male sexual organs, including chronically hard testicles. Mixed with **Saw Palmetto berries,** this herb
is said to reduce an enlarged prostate. **Thuja** is a tonic medicine for the entire reproductive system.

Wild Thyme *(Thymus serpyllum)* has an antiseptic action,
works specifically on the reproductive organs, and is used for
"overly active" people in the "treatment of nervous diseases arising from disturbances in the sexual areas." As Hilda Leyel, the
great English herbalist, goes on to say in a rather euphemistic
way, **Wild Thyme** is used beneficially as a medicine by men and
women who have had a "wild time."

The Chinese use other herbs as well for the male reproductive system including **Asparagus, Licorice, Cattails, Lotus,**
Mugwort, Wild Yam, and **Echinops.**

Chapter 14

Herbal Formulas for Men

Cryptorchism

Cryptorchism or non-descent of the testes is occasionally found in newborn babies. In my own son this condition was tentatively diagnosed at birth, and he was examined on a regular basis until he was six years old. It was thought that my son had only one testicle, but from the time he was three he would tell me that he had two, only one was real small and "hiding." An undescended testicle heats up in the abdominal cavity and can deteriorate and become cancerous. The Oriental treatment consists of acupuncture begun at puberty, and then if the testicle does not descend, herbs are given to "dissolve" it entirely. The Occidental treatment is very much the same except a drug is given to stimulate the descent of the testis. If this does not work, the testis is surgically brought down, or if damaged, it is removed.

My treatment began with an herbal mixture that stimulated the testicle to enlarge it enough to be felt. When I was positive there actually was one (partly due to my little boy's continued assertion that there was a little one "up there hiding"), we proceeded with the surgery to bring it down and to tie it into place. I am glad he had enough self-knowledge to "see" what was going on in his body.

The herbal formula I used included the following herbs:

1 oz each of **Motherwort tops, Helonias,* Sarsaparilla root, Alfalfa tops,** and **Parsley roots and tops**

2 oz each of **Raspberry leaf, Ginseng root,** and **Fenugreek seeds**

½ oz each of **Orange peel, Wild Yam root,** and **Angelica tops**

¼ oz each of **Black Cohosh** and **Cayenne fruits**

The herbs are mixed together and half of the formulation is ground into powder. Stuff the powder into size 00 gelatin capsules. Two should be taken by the young boy (between the ages of six and ten) twice a day for no longer than a month.

Put the other half of the mixture into a green glass bottle and add alcohol (or Crema de Damiana) to barely cover the herbs. Steep at least ten days until the alcohol completely extracts the essence of the herbs. Then draw off the alcohol tincture totally. The dose is ten drops three times per day along with the capsules.

This herbal mixture should stimulate the testicle to descend either temporarily or permanently. If it descends only temporarily, I recommend surgery within a year.

Epididymitis

This inflammation in the epididymis can be treated with the **YEGG Formula;** teas of **Mullein flowers, Lemon Verbena leaves,** and **Comfrey leaves;** a sitz bath that includes **clay, Comfrey root,** and **Marjoram herb;** and **Aloe Vera gel** applied topically if there is an itch.

***Helonias,** another name for **False Unicorn root,** *Chamaelirium luteum.*

A friend took these herbal formulations some years ago when antibiotics prescribed by an allopathic physician were not working. His case history in his own words follows:

First week of February, began to experience dull pain in right testicle, and fearing VD, began sexual abstinence. Four weeks later, pain was rather intense, especially when standing or walking, and testicle had swollen to perhaps twice normal size, and was quite hard and inflamed. Large doses of vitamins C, E ,and others did little good, and pain made sleeping difficult.

Went to see allopathic MD in the second week, and he diagnosed Epididymitus [sic] (infection of the epididium, [sic] a small collecting gland [sic] that lies over and behind each testicle), and prescribed ampicillin, 500 mg. q.i.d.

Took these pills regularly for one week, and there was absolutely no change in the condition, and also, under his advice, began wearing a supporter day and night.

After 7 days of the ampicillin, went to see herbalist, who prescribed a mixture of Ginseng, Echinacea, Golden Seal and Yellow Dock powders, and, not being able to procure gelatin capsules, I took one-half teaspoon q.i.d., along with the ampicillin, which I had had refilled.

The morning after the first day of herbs, there seemed some slight improvement, though not enough to be certain. By the following day (I began the herbs on Friday afternoon, and by Sunday morning) there was definite improvement, the swelling being palpably less severe, and the pain diminished. Five days after beginning the herbs, was able to walk without pain, The swollen gland was down to almost normal size, though still quite hard.

The first 5 days, also boiled an infusion of Comfrey, Echinacea, and Mullein herbs given by the herbalist, and added the infusion to very hot bathwater, in which I would soak for an hour, two or three times a day. Had been soaking also under the MD's advice, but in plain hot water.

By one week after beginning the herbs, the situation was well in hand, and healing proceeded after this time, though gland was not normal until at least a month later, and still (June) has a small hard spot within it, but there has been no recurrence.

The difference between the ampicillin and herbal treatment was startling, and while I admit that the accumulation of penicillin may have begun to work just when the herbs were taken, or that psychological effects were observed, nevertheless, there had been no progress whatsoever until the use of the herbs had begun, and progress immediately thereafter.

Lack of Erection or Impotence

If there is no physiological reason for this condition then try a change of diet and moderate your lifestyle. Use the alkaline food diet: 70% vegetables, fruits, salad, and Potatoes, with the balance of the food being organically grown chicken or turkey or deep-water ocean fish and seafoods. Delete Coffee, pleasure drugs, nicotine, and alcohol from the diet. Add about 100 mg zinc per day plus a **Saw Palmetto** formula. These simple changes alone should cure most cases. Men should also be aware that many drugs inhibit erections, such as those prescribed for high blood pressure, tranquilizers, some medicines used by diabetics, and other drugs. If after changing and simplifying the diet there is still a problem, then seek help from a sex counselor or psychologist.

The mineral supplement zinc plays a very important role in sexual development. It is essential for the production of testosterone in the body. Even a slightly deficient zinc supply in the male body can lead to sexual dysfunction, impotence, and lack of sexual vigor. Heavy smokers and drinkers in particular need more zinc because cadmium, a toxic heavy metal in smoke, interferes with zinc metabolism. Alcohol causes a greater demand for zinc in the body, and I suspect that drugs such as cocaine and marijuana do also. Zinc occurs naturally in seafoods, meats, and eggs.

A Chinese Formula for Impotence

Prepare a 300-cc decoction made from of the following herbs:

8 gm *Selinum monnieri* seeds
7 gm *Epimedium macranthum* leaves
7 gm *Achyranthes bidentata* root
7 gm *Cimicifuga foetida* root
(this is a plant in the same genus as **Black Cohosh**)
5 gm *Dioscorea sativa* root
(related to the Mexican Wild Yam)
6 gm *Acanthopanax spinosum* root epidermis
10 gm *Asparagus lucidus*

The dose is 100 cc three times per day.

Orchitis

Orchitis is an infection of the testis often caused by a virus. The treatment consists of massive doses of vitamin C, 1 gram taken hourly, and the same herbal treatments used for epididymitis. In addition the Chinese use **Nepeta Japonica,** 5 gm of the powdered herb taken daily. Apply the juice of the fresh root of **Turnip, Rutabaga,** or **Radish** topically. If the juice is irritating, dilute it with an equal portion of **Apple Cider Vinegar.**

Prostate Health and Troubles

Treat prostate infections and problems with vitamin supplements, dietary changes, lifestyle changes, and a few simple herbal teas. **Sunflower seeds,** eaten regularly, not only reduce a person's need to smoke, but are important for the health of the prostate. Many cultures swear by the use of **Sunflower seeds** to heal the prostate. Zinc supplements and vitamin C also keep the prostate healthy. High-fat diets seem partially to blame for the enormous number of men suffering from prostate problems. A simple change to the alkaline-forming diet of 70 percent veggies, fruits, and Potatoes seems logical, and much simpler than undergoing surgery or developing cancer.

Any of the herbal remedies that are of value for bladder infections will help heal the prostate. A mixture of **Bearberry leaves, Boneset, Burdock root, Juniper berries, Horsetail,** and **Saw Palmetto berries** is especially good. Mix and store equal parts of the herbs. 1 T of the mixture infused for five minutes in one cup of boiled water is taken twice a day, daily. **Thuja** and **Saw Palmetto berries,** both powdered and stuffed into size 00 gelatin capsules, can be taken 2–3 at a time, twice a day.

Scrotal Eczema

This can be treated with a dusting powder of **Calamus root** or **Cattails.** You can also use applications of **Tea Tree oil** as well as **terpene-free Lavender oil.**

Spermatorrhea

Spermatorrhea is an excessive emission of semen without orgasm. This can be treated with ¼ ounce of the following combination of powdered herbs taken in capsule form daily until the condition subsides:

Mix together the dried and powdered herbs of:
½ oz **Ginseng root**	½ oz **Asparagus root**
½ oz **Licorice root**	½ oz **Ginseng root**
1 oz **Rehmannia**	1¼ oz **Cork tree**

Another useful mixture of herbs is the following tincture.

Use equal quantities of **Lotus root, Cattails,** and **Onion.**

Take ten drops three times per day.

Other herbs that can be taken in tea or as capsules include **Mugwort, Poria,** and **Wild Yam root.**

Venereal Diseases

These are best treated first by a physician with antibiotics, and you may then use detoxifying herbal formulations to bring the body back to optimal health.

The Chinese use the following mixture of herbs in a decoction:

> 5 gms each of **Motherwort**
> root of *Imperata cylindrica* (a perennial grass)
> root of *Phragmites communis* (a perennial marsh grass)
> pitch of *Juncus effusus* (a bog rush)
> **Plantain**
> **Carnation flowers**
> Chenopodium *Kochia scoparia*
> spores of the fern *Lycodium japonicum*
> root of *Echinops dahuricus*
> **Dandelion root**

Add five grams of each herb to 600 cc of water. Make a decoction. The dose is 100 cc three times per day.

Venereal Warts and Herpes

These are quite literally a pain. They can be treated by adopting a more moderate sexual lifestyle, adding 8–10 grams of vitamin C and 50 mg of Zinc to the daily supplements, and applying a concentrated solution of **Mugwort** and **Aloe vera** topically as often as possible throughout the day. It may also help to apply small dabs of **Cayenne pepper in Castor oil,** although this is much less effective for women than for men.

Direct applications of essential oil, such as **Tea Tree** and **Thuja** (see note page 56), have also been found to be useful. Lysine (an amino acid) is good for herpes too.

Herbal Aphrodisiacs

An aphrodisiac must be something that induces sexual excite-ment or prolongs sexual excitement or stimulates sexual excite-ment where none previously existed, or enables the penis to become engorged and stay that way. Or it can be a combination of these elements.

There are many herbs that have been used as aphrodisiacs through the ages. Generally, these herbs were rare or unusual or shaped like a penis or gave the impression of labial lips. Some of these herbs include **Korean ginseng, Coriander, Cardamom, Saw Palmetto berries, Damiana, Sarsaparilla, Gotu Kola, Yohimbe, Muira-puama, Jasmine flowers,** and **Orange buds.** Years ago when I had an herbal cosmetics company called New Age Creations I made a mixture of all these herbs as a tea. I sold many, many pounds of it and still to this day have requests for it. Many letters were sent to me regarding the results obtained from drinking this mixture, and all those comments were positive.

Aphrodisiac Tea

Use herbs that have been cut and sifted or are in powdered form.

> Mix together 1 part each of **Korean ginseng, Saw Palmetto berries, Damiana, Sarsaparilla, Gotu Kola, Yohimbe, Muira-puama,** and ½ part each of **Coriander, Cardamom, Jasmine flowers,** and **Orange buds.**

Add 1 ounce of the mixed herbs to 1 quart of water. Bring to a boil and simmer for 10 minutes. Turn off heat and infuse. Drink 1 cup night and morning and either hot or cold for at least 3 days prior to need. Naturally, it would be helpful if you encouraged your sex partner to do the same.

Part III

HELPFUL INFORMATION

Glossary of Herbs
Herbs for the Reproductive System
Acid-Alkaline Diet and Chart
Simple Methods of Preparation
Glossary of Terms
Source List

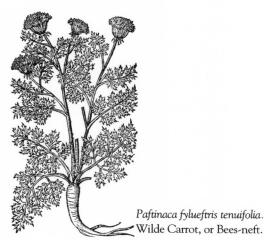

Paftinaca fylueftris tenuifolia.
Wilde Carrot, or Bees-neft.

Notes

Glossary of Herbs

The common and Latin names for the *main herbs* used to treat men and women.

Achillea millefolium — *Yarrow*

Alchemilla vulgaris — Lady's Mantle

Aletris farinosa — Unicorn root or Star root

Angelica atropurpurea or *A. sinensis* or *A. archangelica* — Angelica or Dong Quai

Aralia racemosa — American Spikenard

Aristolochia clematitis — Birthwort

Artemisia vulgaris — Mugwort

Caulophyllum thalictroides — Blue Cohosh, Squaw root, Papoose root

Chamaelirium luteum — False Unicorn root (*Helonias dioica*)

Cimicifuga racemosa — Black Cohosh

Cnicus benedictus — Blessed Thistle

Cypripedium pubescens — Lady's Slipper

Daucus carota — Carrot

Dioscorea villosa — Mexican Wild Yam and Wild Yam

Epimedium spp. — Barrenwort

Glycyrrhiza glabra, *G. lepidota* — Licorice and Wild Licorice

Gossypium herbaceum — Cotton Root

Helonias dioica — False Unicorn root (*Chamaelirium luteum*)

Humulus lupulus — Hops

Illicium verum — Star Anise

Mentha pulegium — Pennyroyal

Mitchella repens — Squaw Vine

Ocimum basilicum — Basil

Oenothera biennis — Evening Primrose or Kings Plant

Panax quinquefolius, *P. ginseng* — American Ginseng, Korean Ginseng

Petroselinum crispum — Parsley

Rosa spp. — Rose

Rosmarinus officinalis — Rosemary

Rubus idaeus, and other ssp. — Raspberry and Red Raspberry

Ruta graveolens — Rue

Salix caprea — Pussy Willow

Sassafras officinale — Sassafras

Silybum marianum — Holy Thistle

Smilax ssp. — Sarsaparilla

Stillingia sylvatica — Stillingia or Queen's Root

Trillium erectum — Bethroot or Birthroot

Turnera diffusa — Damiana

Urtica dioica — Nettle

Viburnum opulus — Crampbark, Guelder Rose

Vitex agnus-castus, *Agnus-castus* — Life Root, Life Plant, Chaste Tree

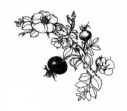

Herbs for the Reproductive System

Alfalfa
Medicago sativa

Used during pregnancy, as its rich nutritional content makes it a valuable food.
SEE Pregnancy & Childbirth

Agnus Castus
Vitus Agnus Castus
Chaste Tree
aka Life Plant,
Life Root

Relieves premenstrual water retention and hormonally induced acne.
SEE Menstrual Regulation Formula, Estrogen Tea Formula, Progesterone Tea Formula, Menopause Tea Formula 2

American Spikenard
Aralia racemosa

The root is used as tea for women in labor to quicken childbirth and ease pain.

Angelica
Angelica atropurpurea
Angelica archangelica
Angelica sinensis
aka Dong Quai

SEE Menstrual Regulation Formula, Estrogen Tea Formula

Anise seed
Pimpinella anisum

SEE Pregnancy & Childbirth

Apricot Kernels
Prunus armeniaca

SEE General Formula for Menstrual Tardiness

Barrenwort
Epimedium ssp.

Not often used.

Basil
Ocimum basilicum

Antispasmodic.
SEE Pregnancy & Childbirth

Bearberry
Arctostaphylos uva-ursi

Gives strength and tone to all the urinary passages.
Used as a tea for a healthy prostate.

Bethroot
Trillium erectum
aka Birthroot

Antiseptic tonic expectorant, used in hemorrhages and to promote childbirth.

Birthwort
Aristolochia clematitis

A European plant sometimes considered an abortifacient.

Black Cohosh
Cimicifuga racemosa

Prepares uterus for birth, makes labor less difficult, relieves uterine distress during birthing.
Strongly affects the nervous system.
Used in any formula treating erection problems.
SEE Pregnancy & Childbirth, Menopause Tea Formula 1

Black Horehound
Ballota nigra

Uterine tonic.

Black Willow
Salix nigra

Anaphrodisiac and a sedative tonic for the reproductive organs.

Blessed Thistle
Cnicus benedictus

SEE Menstrual Regulation Formula, Progesterone Tea Formula, Pregnancy & Childbirth, Menopause Tea Formulas 1 & 2

Blue Cohosh
Caulophyllum thalictroides
aka Papoose Root,
Squaw Root

Used to prolong the pregnancy until the fetus is properly developed, and after childbirth.
SEE Pregnancy & Childbirth, Menopause

Boneset
Eupatorium purpureum

Used for irritation in the urinary passage.

Buchu Leaves
Agathosma ssp.

SEE Cystitis Tea Formula

Burdock
Arctium lappa

Seed and leaf powdered for use in scrotal eczema, taken internally for *prostatitis, epididymitis*. Root used by Chinese in alternative treatments of *syphilis* externally on chronic sores. Used for uterine displacements.
SEE Bolus Formula

Carrot
Daucus carota

SEE General Formula for Menstrual Tardiness

Catnip
Nepeta cataria

Antispasmodic. Used for morning sickness.
SEE Pregnancy & Childbirth

Cattails
Typha angustifolia

Root used as an astringent.

Chamomile
Chamaemelum nobile
Matricaria recutita

Antispasmodic. Used for morning sickness.
SEE Pregnancy & Childbirth
SEE *The Aromatherapy Book*

Chickweed
Stellaria media

SEE Basic Bolus Formula for vaginal infections

Clover tops
Trifolium pratense

May be used in pregnancy.
SEE Pregnancy & Childbirth

Comfrey leaves and root
Symphytum officinale

Aid in protein synthesis, encourage milk production.
SEE Bolus for vaginal infections, Cystitis Tea Formula, Pregnancy & Childbirth, Menopause Tea Formula 2, Basic Formula for Cleansing Douche

Cornsilk
Zea mays

Used for inflamed urinary passages.
SEE Formula for Inflamed Urinary Passages

Cotton Root
Gossypium herbaceum

Abortifacient.

Couch Grass
Elymus repens

SEE Cystitis Tea Formula

Cowslip
Primula veris

Has been used as a tea and a douche for uterine tumors, and as a mild sedative.

Cramp bark
Viburnum opulus
aka Highbush
Cranberry

Antispasmodic for menstrual cramps.

Damiana
Turnera diffusa

A general stimulant and sexual tonic.

Echinacea Root
Echinacea angustifolia

Stimulates the immune system.
SEE Formula for Uterine Infection, Bolus for Vaginal Infection, Cystitis Tea Formula

Evening Primrose
Oenothera biennis
aka Kings Plant

SEE General Formula for Menstrual
Tardiness, Pregnancy & Childbirth

False Unicorn Root
Chamaelirium luteum
Helonias dioica

SEE Menopause Tea Formulas
1 & 2

Fennel seed
Foeniculum vulgare

Used as a galactogogue.
SEE Pregnancy & Childbirth

Garlic cloves
Allium sativum

Antibacterial, antifungal, antiviral.
SEE Vaginal Infections Formula

Ginger Root
Zingiber officinale

SEE YEGG Formula for vaginal
infection

Ginseng, American
aka Korean Ginseng
Panax quinquefolius
Panax schinseng

Used for thousands of years in the
East as a medicine for the lymphatic
and reproductive systems. Increases
erection ability, retards impotence.
Incompatible with iron
supplements and black tea.
SEE Progesterone Tea Formula,
YEGG Formula for Vaginal
Infections, Menopause Tea
Formulas 1 & 2

Golden Seal
Hydrastis canadensis

Used as a douche for infection,
taken internally as an antibacterial,
antiviral, antifungal.
SEE YEGG Formula for Vaginal
Infections, Bolus Douche for
Vaginal Infections, Cystitis Tea For-
mula, Basic Formula for Cleansing
Douche

Groundsel
Senecio vulgaris

Used widely in treatment of male sexual organ.

Guelder Rose
Viburnum opulus
aka Highbush
Cranberry

Used as a uterine sedative.
SEE Pregnancy & Childbirth
SEE also Cramp bark

Helonias Dioica

SEE False Unicorn Root

Holy Thistle
Silybum marianum

Liver tonic.

Hops
Humulus lupulus

Antispasmodic.
SEE Pregnancy & Childbirth.

Juniper Berries
Juniperus communis

Diuretic and carminative.
SEE Cystitis Tea

Lady's Mantle
Alchemilla vulgaris

Astringent. Used for excessive menstruation and for general bleeding.

Lady's Slipper
Cypripedium pubescens

This plant is being overpicked—probably should no longer be used. Formerly for muscle spasms and anxiety.

Lavender
Lavandula angustifolia

Used in birthing tea.
SEE Pregnancy & Childbirth

Licorice Root
Glycyrrhiza glabra
Glycyrrhiza lepidota

SEE Menstrual Regulation Formula, Estrogen Tea Formula, Menopause Tea Formulas 1 & 2

Lobelia
Lobelia inflata

Used to subdue spasm.
SEE Pregnancy & Childbirth

Lotus root
Nelumbo lutea

Used as a cleansing vaginal douche.
Eaten as a female tonic food.

Marjoram herb
Origanum majorana

Used for certain uterine tumors, and helps to regulate the cycle when used as a douche to bring on menses *(emmenagogue)*.

Marshmallow Root
Althaea officinalis

SEE Bolus Formula for Vaginal Infection, Cystitis Tea Formula, Pregnancy & Childbirth

(Mexican) Wild Yam
Dioscorea villosa

Synthesized for birth control.
SEE Menopause Tea Formula 2

Mistletoe leaves
(not berries)
Phoradendron serotinum
(Amer.) and
Viscum album (Eur.)

Smooth muscle stimulant for uterus and circulation. Antispasmodic. SEE Pregnancy & Childbirth

Motherwort
Leonurus cardiaca

Has a soothing effect on the uterus, relieving nervous disorders in this organ.

Mugwort leaves
Artemisia vulgaris

Menstrual stimulant.

Muira-puama Root
Liriosma ovata

Aphrodisiac and nerve stimulant.

Mullein Flowers
Verbascum thapsis

SEE Pregnancy & Childbirth

Myrtle leaves
Myrtus communis

Stimulates the mucous secretions of the vagina. Used as a drinking tea and as a douche. Excellent douche on the last day of menses because of its lovely aroma. Helps relieve pubescent cramps. Regulates the cycle. Increases secretions in men with a diminution of sexual fluids.

Nettle tops
Urtica dioica

Contains easily assimilable iron.
SEE Pregnancy & Childbirth

Nutmeg kernels
Myristica fragrans

Used in birthing tea.
SEE Pregnancy & Childbirth

Oats
Avena sativa

Used in connection with Tree of
Life to stimulate the nerves.

Parsley (roots, leaves, seeds)
Petroselinum crispum

SEE General Formula for
Menstrual Tardiness, Cystitis Tea

Pasque Flower
aka Wind Flower
Pulsatilla vulgaris

Encourages the secretions of the
body. Used to treat inflammation
of the testis and inflammation of
the prostate (*orchitis prostatitis*).

Peach Leaf & kernels
Prunus persica

Prevents nausea.
SEE Pregnancy & Childbirth

Pennyroyal tops
Mentha pulegium

Taken in small doses, helps regulate
the cycle and soothe spasmodic
contractions of the uterus. In larger
doses, causes "natural" abortion.
SEE General Formula for Menstrual
Tardiness, Cystitis Tea

Peony Root
Paeonia officinalis

Emmenagogue.
SEE Estrogen Tea

Peppermint herb
Mentha x piperita

Antispasmodic. Used for morning
sickness.
SEE Pregnancy & Childbirth

Peyotl tops
Lophophora williamsii

SEE Pregnancy & Childbirth

Plantain tops
Plantago major

Contain potash.
SEE Pregnancy & Childbirth

Pussy Willow
Salix caprea

Anaphrodisiac, sexual sedative.

Queen's Root
(Queen's Delight)
Stillingia sylvatica
aka Stillingia

Diuretic, fresh root chewed for
leucorrhea. Influences secretory
action.

Red Clover tops
Trifolium pratense

SEE Menstrual Regulation Formula,
Estrogen Tea Formula, Menopause
Tea Formula 2

(Red) Raspberry Leaf
Rubus idaeus
Rubus stringosus

Antispasmodic, tones uterine
muscle. Contains fragarine, a
uterine relaxant. Used as tea during
pregnancy and lactation. SEE
Progesterone Tea, Pregnancy &
Childbirth

Rhododendron flowers
Rhododendron spp.

Flower effective in treating a
hydrocele, a collection of fluid other
than blood or pus in the scrotum.
SEE Poultice for Scrotum.

Rose petal and hips
Rosa spp.

Hips have vitamin C.
Rose petal tea is a female tonic.

Rose Geranium Oil
Pelargonium spp.

SEE Formula To Get Rid of Fibroid
Tumors in One Week, Cysts

Rosemary
Rosmarinus officinalis

SEE PMT, Acne & Water
Retention, Menopause Tea
Formula 2

Rue leaves
Ruta graveolens

SEE Pregnancy & Childbirth

Sarsaparilla root
Smilax spp.

SEE Menstrual Regulation Formula,
Progesterone Tea Formula,
Menopause Tea Formulas 1 & 2

Sassafras bark & root
Sassafras officinale

Aromatic stimulant, sometimes used as an abortifacient.

Saw Palmetto berries
Serenoa repens

A general stimulant and sexual tonic.
SEE Male Reproductive Organs Formula

Slippery Elm inner bark
Ulmus fulva

SEE the Bolus Formula for vaginal infection

Spikenard root
Aralia racemosa

SEE Menopause Tea Formulas 1 & 2

Squaw Vine
Mitchella repens

SEE Bolus Formula for Vaginal Infection, Pregnancy & Childbirth

Star Anises
Illicium verum

Aromatic.

Tansy tops
Tanacetum vulgare

SEE Pregnancy & Childbirth

Thuja leaves or oil

SEE Cysts
SEE Tree of Life

Tree of Life
Thuja occidentalis
aka Arbor Vitae

Used to treat chronically hard testicles. Tonic for the entire reproductive system.

True Unicorn Root
Aletris farinosa
aka Star Root

SEE Menopause Formula 2

Uva Ursi tops
Arctostaphylos uva-ursi
(Folia—*Ericacaea* family)

SEE Cystitis Tea, Pregnancy & Childbirth

Wild Celery
seeds & tops
Apium graveolens

SEE Pregnancy & Childbirth

Wild Thyme herb
Thymus spp.

Used for nervous disorders arising from any problem in the reproductive organs. Used to treat "disturbances in the sexual areas" by people who have had a "wild time." Has an antiseptic action.

Yarrow tops
Achillea millefolium

SEE Pregnancy & Childbirth

Yellow Dock Root
Rumex crispus

Natural antibiotic, considered a powerful alterative.
SEE YEGG Formula, Basic Bolus, Douche for Vaginal Infection, Basic Formula for Cleansing Douche

Yoghurt
Lactobacillus acidophilus

SEE Vaginal Infection

Note: Source for plants, names, and correct spelling: D. J. Mabberley, *The Plant Book* (Cambridge, MA: Cambridge University Press, 1989).

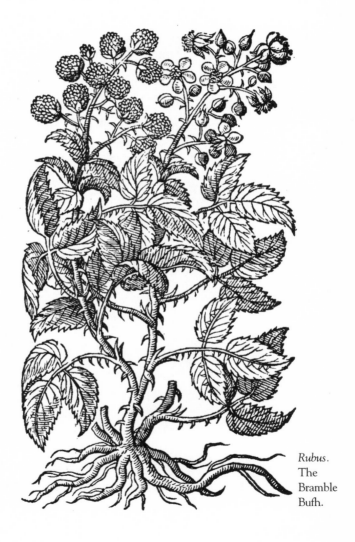

Rubus.
The
Bramble
Bufh.

Acid-Alkaline Diet and Chart

The Acid-Alkaline Diet is the key to rational, scientific eating. You need not study food chemistry or worry about what you eat if you follow these instructions and the chart on the following page.

Science has divided foods, like chemicals, into two classes: alkaline-forming, or practically safe foods, and acid-forming, or somewhat dangerous ones. If you eat more than 80% alkaline foods, mainly fruits and vegetables (rich in organic mineral salts and vitamins), thus preserving the normal alkalinity of the blood, you need not think about diets. This is the key to all balancing of foods for you. Remember always to eat plenty of these health-promoting items, especially when you do eat acid-formers, such as meat, cheese, nuts, grains, etc. Because these items are acid-forming is no reason to exclude them entirely—but use them judiciously and in correct balance, so they will yield the greatest good.

Gland tone means perfect health. Glands feed mainly upon body secretions, and the healthy body must have living mineral and alkaline elements in the main. Fruits should predominate at breakfast. For lunch, fruit or vegetables with a possible alkaline dairy product. At dinner, vegetables, especially salads. Use cereal products sparingly; proteins, fats, sweets, moderately. Have only whole-grain goods. I prefer eating a protein at lunchtime (such as sashimi or chicken to keep me awake), and carbohy-drates like pasta with a simple vegetable or herb sauce (Pasta al Pesto at dinner) to relax me and help me sleep.

Fruits are not really laxative; they merely help produce diges-tive juices which promote good elimination, while their high water content keeps the bowels moist and soft, really a normal condition. Protein, starch, sugar, and fats leave acid reactions. Thus an alkaline diet diminishes acidity of the urine by neu-tralizing and absorbing normal body acids. It also forms a reserve of bicarbonates, which help to maintain neutrality; you are aid-ing your body to overcome the bad effects of acid foods you do eat. The only other food knowledge you need is harmonious combination, which is available in any modern health work.

The average person can be safe on an 80–20% by weight proportion. Watch yourself. Plan your meals to follow this valu-able acid-alkaline chart, the most complete, simple, and up-to-date in existence. However, don't make a fetish of this, but observe it in a rational manner. Even if you do eat an all-acid meal, make your next two or three all-alkaline, and don't worry about it!

Lastly, to maintain a perfect condition, observe general health rules. Rest and sleep are alkalizers. So is exercise, fresh air, plea-sure, laughter, conversation, enjoyment—even love! Acidifiers are worry, fear, anger, gossip, hatred, envy, "crabbing," selfish-ness, and silence—also love-hunger. Health to you!

Acid-Alkaline Chart

Key:

VERY ALKALINE	AL	VERY ACID	AC
Slightly Alkaline	al	Acid	ac

Proteins

SOYBEANS	AL
RAW MILK, NONFAT	AL
buttermilk	ac
cottage cheese	ac
yogurt	ac
eggs	ac
cheeses	ac
yeast	ac
raw milk, whole	ac
fish	ac
fowl	ac
meat of any sort	AC

Vegetables   AL

ALL VEGETABLES ARE
ALKALINE *except*

asparagus	ac
artichoke	ac
Jerusalem artichokes	ac

Melons   AL

ALL MELONS ARE
ALKALINE

Seeds & Nuts

ALMONDS	AL
other seeds & nuts	acid

Sugars, Fats & Oils

HONEY	AL
OLIVE OIL	AL
SOY OIL	AL
CORN OIL	AL
AVOCADO OIL	AL
sunflower oil	ac
sesame oil	ac
brown sugar	ac
white sugar	ac
milk sugar	ac
maple syrup	ac
cane syrup	ac
malt syrup	ac
blackstrap molasses	ac
butter & margarine	ac
cream	ac
all nut oils	ac

Carbohydrates

LIMA BEANS	AL
PARSNIPS	AL
CORN	AL
POTATOES	AL
(WHITE OR SWEET)	
MILLET	AL
BUCKWHEAT	AL
sprout bread (made only with sprouts)	al

dried split peas	ac	ELDERBERRIES	AL
beans of any kind	ac	FIGS	AL
bread	ac	GOOSEBERRIES	AL
rice, brown or white	ac	GRAPES	AL
lentils	ac	GUAVAS	AL
cereals	ac	HUCKLEBERRIES	AL
chestnuts	ac	MANGOS	AL
peanuts	ac	NECTARINES	AL
oats	ac	PAPAYAS	AL
wheat	ac	PEACHES	AL
rye	AC	PEARS	AL
barley	ac	PERSIMMON	AL
dhal	ac	PINEAPPLE	AL
aduki	ac	PLUMS	AL
cashews	ac	POMEGRANATES	AL
		QUINCE	AL
Herbs & Roots	AL	RASPBERRIES	AL
IN GENERAL, ALL ARE		RHUBARB	AL
ALKALINE		DRIED FRUITS	AL
		CITRUS FRUITS	AL
Fruits		tomatoes	al
		blueberries	ac
APPLES	AL	cranberries	ac
APRICOTS	AL	currants	ac
BANANAS	AL	kumquats	ac
BLACKBERRIES	AL	loganberries	ac
CACTUS	AL	loquat	ac
CHERRIES	AL	strawberries	ac
COCONUT	AL	sour fruits	ac
DATE	AL	pickled fruits	ac

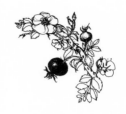

Simple Methods of Preparation

There are many methods one can use to administer herbal medicines and many modes of preparation. Each of these methods and preparations can be performed in many different ways, some of which I have described in other works. There is no best method. Twenty years ago, when I first started making herbal infusions, I used the standard directions that I had seen in many books: heat the water, and steep ten to twenty minutes. Now my method of preparing an infusion is quite different and neither the original nor my modernized version is "better."

Water Formulas

Tea (beverage). Warm pot, boil 1 cup water. Pour boiling water over approximately 1 tablespoon of herbs, cover and *steep* 3–5 minutes. With more herbs and longer steeping this becomes an infusion and therefore more medicinal.

Tisane (also Barley Water or Ptisan). A nourishing decoction or infusion, which often has a slight medicinal quality, originally made from Barley. Now frequently used for a beverage tea made from flowers. Can also be defined as an infusion of herbs.

Infusion. An infusion usually involves the soft parts of the plant, such as the herb, leaf, or flower, 1 ounce of which is soaked or "infused" for 10–20 minutes in up to 1 quart of just-below-boiling (temperature) water. Simmer the herbs a moment or two and then infuse them.

Decoction. A decoction is usually made of the hard parts of the plant, such as the root, bark, or seed—the tougher parts. Put 1 ounce of herb and 20 ounces of water into a pot. Bring to a boil an simmer for 10–20 minutes or longer. Steep, strain, and drink. If making decoction of both hard and soft parts, boil the hard parts (such as the bark and seeds) and add the soft parts (such as the herb or flower) during the steeping cycle.

Oil and Wax Formulas

Ointment. A medicinal ointment is simply an herb crisped in lard, strained, cooled, and stored. This constitutes a "simple." Simmer 1 ounce of the herb in 4 ounces of lard (or Crisco, or whatever) in a nonmetal pot, preferably a double boiler, for 10–30 minutes. Strain and cool. Different simples may be mixed for different effects.

Cerate. Use a single herb or a mixture of herbs. The mixture of herbs depends on the effects desired. Cerates are also cosmetic creams. Simmer 1 ounce of herbs in 8 ounces of oil plus 1 ounce of wine until the wine is boiled off. Strain off the herbs and add ½ ounce solidifier (beeswax or lanolin), heat only until everything is incorporated, remove from heat, and beat with a wooden spoon or whisk until cool.

Direct Applications

Plaster. A plaster is usually a macerated, bruised bunch of fresh hot herbs placed between 2 sheets of muslin and applied to the aching or bruised area, or to the chest for respiratory problems. This causes increased circulation and sweating which cleanses the system of impurities, lowers fever, and reduces swelling.

Poultice. Same as plaster, except the herbs are applied directly and a hot cloth wrapped around to keep them hot. Used to open a dirty sore or abscess.

Sitz Bath. A sitz bath is a shallow bath that one sits in to soothe aching or sore vaginal or anal parts. An herbal sitz bath is simply an infusion of herbs and water, strained or unstrained.

For the Future

Elixir. Infuse 4 ounces of herbs in 4 ounces or more boiling water for 10 minutes or longer. Add 8 ounces of 100-proof vodka. Strain off the herbs through a silk cloth and squeeze out the liquid completely. Set aside the squeezed herbs for other uses. You can also add a sweetener to the elixir (liquid) for taste. Honey will act as a natural preservative. Take a spoonful or so every hour like cough syrup. A child should take a teaspoonful every 4 hours.

Mellite. 1 ounce herb, 20 ounces water. Simmer 20 minutes. Strain, and add 4 or more ounces of honey.

To Preserve

Tincture. Tinctures are very concentrated solutions that can be added to teas and infusions or diluted for use in cosmetic or medicinal preparations. They can be kept for long periods in a very small place. A tincture is a solution of medicinal substances in alcohol, preserved by maceration, digestion, or percolation. Herbs whose active ingredients have been extracted by alcohol are also called tinctures. The advantage of alcohol over water (as in a tea or infusion) is that alcohol dissolves some substances that are sparingly or not at all soluble in water. Another advantage is that alcohol is a preservative. The disadvanage, of course, is that if you need many herbs at the same time you may ingest too much alcohol.

The time-honored way of making tinctures is as follows: Start with 150 proof (60–80%) alcohol. I use vodka since it generally does not alter the taste of the herbal tincture. Originally, high-proof brandy was used, but brandy taste often does not mix well with herb taste.

Take about 4 ounces of your herb, root, bark, or seed and bruise, slice, or pulverize it. It is best to work with plants in the dry state, as tinctures made with freshly picked plants are not as good. Coarsely ground herbs are better than powdered because the powders often stick together and do not extract well. When making a tincture of several substances use the least soluble first, such as bark, then seed, then herb, and then flower; this allows the different substances to macerate for successively shorter lengths of time depending on their delicacy or lack of it.

Add 2 pints (4 cups) alcohol to the pulverized or coarsely ground herb. Two weeks is the usual amount of time to allow the herb and alcohol to commingle, though the time really depends on the substance. Flowers, for instance, take only a few days to warm and soak (macerate) in the alcohol, while barks may take several months. Shake or stir daily.

When the tincture has taken on the quality of the plant material (scent, color, vitality), strain carefully through several layers of cheesecloth or silk cloth, or press through a hydraulic press.

Store in small lightproof containers in a dark place. Note that the preceding directions are very general and that properly made tinctures are a result of careful work and judgment on the part of the maker. Each plant has its own characteristics — its own scent, time of extraction, and so forth. These must all be taken into account when making tinctures.

Internal Use

Bolus. A bolus is a suppository, used either anally or vaginally, and made by adding a mixture of powdered herbs to enough melted cocoa butter to make a consistency like pie dough. This mixture is then rolled into a pencil shape in wax paper, refrigerated until hard, and then cut into 1-inch sections for later use. The bolus is best applied at night, where the cocoa butter will melt at body temperature, to slowly release the virtues of the herbs. The exact quantity of herbs to cocoa butter is difficult to determine due to the different types of plant materials used, but a reasonable beginning is 2 oz of mixed herbs to ½ oz of melted cocoa butter.

YEGG *Formula*

YEGG Formula™ is a mixture of roots in varying proportions to treat different conditions. **Echinacea root** to fight infection by encouraging the production of white blood cells, **Yellow Dock root** to cleanse the blood, **Golden Seal root** to counteract bacteria and viruses, and **Ginseng root** to encourage the health of the lymphatic system.

YEGG Formula: **Yellow dock root, Echinacea root, Golden seal root,** and **Ginseng root, Ginger root,** or **Garlic.**

YEGG Formula can be formulated for different types of problems, as follows:

YEGG Lymphatic system: 1·2 · 2· 2 (Ginseng)
YEGG Bacterial infection: 1·3 ·3 ·1 (Garlic)
YEGG Immune stimulant: 1·2·2·1 (Ginseng)
YEGG Skin Ailments: 4·3·2·1 (Ginseng)
YEGG Digestive: 1·2 ·1 ·2 (Ginger)

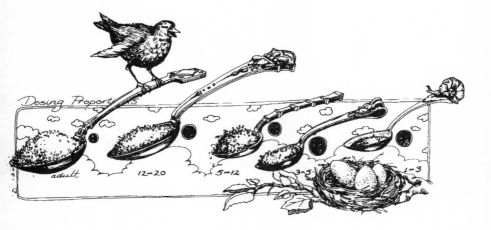

Dosing Proportions

adult   12—20   5—12   3—5   1—3

Notes

Glossary of Terms

Abortifacient: A drug or other agent that induces the expulsion of a fetus.

Alterative: An agent that produces gradual beneficial change in the body, usually by improving nutrition, without having any marked specific effect and without causing sensible evacuation.

Analgesic: A drug that relieves or diminishes pain; anodyne.

Anaphrodisiac: An agent that reduces sexual desire or potency.

Anesthetic: An agent that deadens sensation.

Anthelmintic: An agent that destroys or expels intestinal worms; vermicide; vermifuge.

Anthocyanins: Any of a class of soluble glycoside pigments that are responsible for most of the blue to red colors in leaves, flowers, and other plant parts.

Antibiotic: An agent that destroys or arrests the growth of microorganisms.

Anticoagulant: An agent that prevents clotting in a liquid, as in blood.

Antiemetic: An agent that counteracts nausea and relieves vomiting.

Antihydrotic: An agent that reduces or suppresses perspiration.

Antiperiodic: An agent that counteracts periodic or intermittent diseases (such as malaria).

Antipyretic: An agent that prevents or reduces fever.

Antiseptic: An agent for destroying or inhibiting pathogenic or putrefactive bacteria.

Antispasmodic: An agent that relieves or checks spasms or cramps.

Aperient: A mild stimulant for the bowels, a gentle purgative.

Aphrodisiac: An agent for arousing or increasing sexual desire or potency.

Appetizer: An agent that excites the appetite.

Arbutin: A crystalline glucoside found in the leaves of plants and sometimes used as a urinary antiseptic.

Aromatic: A substance having an agreeable odor and stimulating qualities.

Astringent: An agent that contracts organic tissues, reducing secretions or discharges.

Balsam: 1. A soothing or healing agent. 2. A resinous substance obtained from the exudations of various trees and used in medicinal preparations.

Bitter: Characterized by a bitter principle that acts on the mucous membranes of the mouth and stomach to increase appetite and promote digestion.

Calmative: An agent that has a mild sedative or tranquilizing effect.

Cardiac: An agent that stimulates or otherwise affects the heart.

Carminative: An agent for expelling gas from the intestines.

Cathartic: An agent that acts to empty the bowels; laxative.

Cholagogue: An agent for increasing the flow of bile into the intestines.

Coagulant: An agent that induces clotting in a liquid, as in blood.

Counterirritant: An agent for producing irritation in one part of the body to counteract irritation or inflammation in another part.

Cystitis: Inflammation of the urinary bladder. It is accompanied by pain and frequency of urination.

Demulcent: A substance that soothes irritated tissue, particularly mucous membranes.

Deodorant: An herb that has the effect of destroying or masking odors.

Depressant: An agent that lessens nervous or functional activity; opposite of stimulant.

Detergent: An agent that cleanses wounds and sores of diseased or dead matter.

Diaphoretic: An agent that promotes perspiration; sudorific.

Digestive: An agent that promotes or aids digestion.

Diuretic: An agent that increases the secretion and expulsion of urine.

Dysmenorrhea: Menstrual cycle that is painful.

Emetic: An agent that causes vomiting.

Emmenagogue: An agent that promotes menstrual flow.

Emollient: An agent used externally to soften and soothe.

Epididymitis: Inflammation of the epididymis, a structure immediately adjacent to the testicle, often caused by gonorrhea.

Expectorant: An agent that promotes the discharge of mucus from the respiratory passages.

Febrifuge: An agent that reduces or eliminates fever.

Fomentation: Cloths soaked in hot herbal decoctions or infusions and wrung out and applied to sore, infected, or aching areas to reduce inflammation or ease pain.

Graafian follicle: A vesicle in the ovary enclosing a developing egg.

Hemostatic: An agent that stops bleeding.

Hepatic: A drug that acts on the liver.

Hydragogue: A purgative that produces abundant water discharge.

Hypnotic: An agent that promotes or produces sleep.

Infusion: A mixture of herb and water, brought to a boil, removed from the fire, steeped or infused, and used as a drink or an external wash.

Irritant: An agent that causes inflammation or abnormal sensitivity in living tissue.

Lactation: The secretion and yielding of milk by the mammary gland.

Laxative: An agent promoting evacuation of the bowels; a mild purgative.

Macerate: To extract and soften by soaking in a fluid.

Mastitis: Inflammation of a breast.

Mucilaginous: Characterized by a gummy or gelatinous consistency.

Nephritic: A medicine applicable to diseases of the kidney.

Nervine: An agent that has a calming or soothing effect on the nerves; formerly, any agent that acts on the nervous system.

Ovulation: To produce ovules or discharge them from an ovary.

Oxytocic: An agent that stimulates contraction of the uterine muscle and so facilitates or speeds up childbirth.

Pectoral: A remedy for pulmonary or other chest diseases.

Peptide analog: Functions similar to a peptide chain.

Poultice: An application of hot, moist herb or infusion directly to the skin.

Prostatitis: Inflammation of the prostate gland.

Purgative: An agent that produces a vigorous emptying of the bowels.

Putrefaction: Decomposition of tissue as a result of the action of bacteria, such as gangrene.

Restorative: An agent that restores consciousness or normal physiological activity.

Rubefacient: A gentle local irritant that produces reddening of the skin.

Sebaceous gland: The gland in the skin which contains sebum, an oily waxy substance.

Sedative: A soothing agent that reduces nervousness, distress, or irritation.

Sialagogue: An agent that stimulates the secretion of saliva.

Specific: An agent that cures or alleviates a particular condition or disease.

Stimulant: An agent that excites or quickens the activity of physiological processes.

Stomachic: An agent that strengthens, stimulates, or tones the stomach.

Styptic: An agent that contracts tissues; astringent; specifically, a hemostatic agent that stops bleeding by contracting blood vessels.

Sudorific: An agent that promotes or increases perspiration.

Tincture: A strained solution of herbs and alcohol, to be used internally or externally.

Tonic: An agent that strengthens or invigorates organs or the entire organism.

Vasoconstrictor: An agent that widens the blood vessels, thus lowering blood pressure.

Vermicide: An agent that destroys intestinal worms.

Vermifuge: An agent that causes the expulsion of intestinal worms.

Vesicant: An agent that produces blisters.

Vulnerary: A healing application for wounds.

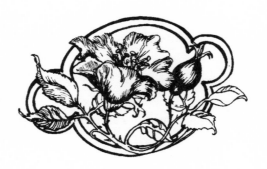

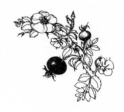

Source List

Aromatherapy & Herbal Studies Course/Herbal Studies Library. 219 Carl Street, San Francisco, CA 94117. The Aromatherapy & Herbal Studies Course is designed and directed by the author, Jeanne Rose. All homework and questions are personally answered by myself. Seventy percent of graduates are working in various herbal fields. The Aromatherapy Course is considered a specialty study and an advanced course.

Send $2.50 for a complete brochure/catalog listing retail and wholesale prices of Jeanne Rose's books, as well as information regarding courses, intensives, and upcoming events.

East Earth Trade Winds, P.O. Box 493151, Redding, CA 96049–3151. A fine listing of Chinese herbs, products, herbal mixtures, supplies, and books. Order toll-free, 24 hours a day: 1–800–258–6878.

Herb Products, 11012 Magnolia Blvd., North Hollywood, CA 91601. What can you say about a company that has been in the same location with the same friendly staff for twenty years or so? And with the same high-quality merchandise—always with reasonable prices. They sell everything herbal, herbs, oils, and other items, including Carrot seeds. No charge for the mail-order catalog. Get it and see!

Herbal BodyWorks, 219 Carl Street, San Francisco, CA 94117. This company went into business in 1965 as New Age Creations, primarily as a clothier making organically designed 100% pure cotton, wool, linen, and silk garments for the rock-and-roll stars of the '60s. By 1968, the business had evolved into "the only real organic, body-care & natural cosmetics on the market. Absolutely pure, natural herbs and oils. NO synthetic scents ... NO chemical preservatives ... NO additives ... Beautiful cosmetics gathered from the earth and good enough to eat" [from an original catalog of products dated September 1973.] The same is true to this day, although the number of products has been greatly reduced.

Also, a new line of "perfect body-care for complete ritual" products called Ritual Works! has been introduced. Each type of product comes in each of the seven colors of the spectrum and has been made with correlating pure essential oil aromas.

Bruise Juice is one of the original products, a medicinal oil that is still being made in the old-fashioned healthful way using organically-grown herbs and enhanced with therapeutic-quality pure essential oils. This product is a formula dating from 1650 which reduces bruising and heals insect bites and plant rashes. Also, Herbal BodyWorks was the first to make aromatherapy products and color therapy-coordinated products, massage oils, and potpourris. $2.50 for catalog.

Indiana Botanic Gardens, P.O. Box 5, Hammond, IN 46325. This has always been one of my favorite herb stores. I have been doing mail-order business with them for twenty years and have never been disappointed. They have a recipe for *real marshmallows* using Marshmallow root. Write for their free catalog and enjoy yourself—plenty of herbal reading to entertain you.

Island Herbs, Waldron Island, WA 98297. Sea plants are their specialty but they also have aromatic Northwest wild-crafted herbs such as Mugwort, Yarrow, and Grindelia. A SASE is needed for the mail-order catalog. I am especially drawn to the naturally-harvested Sea Lettuce, a green seaweed with excellent nourishing properties for your insides and outsides.

Jeanne Rose Aromatherapy, 219 Carl Street, San Francisco, CA 94117. A source for high-quality essential oils that can be hard to find, color therapy bath herbs and rubbing oils, hydrosols, and other body care treatments. Specialty products include four Aromatherapy First Aid Kits™ formulated for Travel & Minor Emergencies, Women's Care, Stress Relief, and Meditation. Each kit contains four pure essential oils and instructions and is packaged in a hand-woven Guatemalan bag, perfect for purse, medicine cabinet, glove box, or travel, and costs $25.00. $2.50 for shipping.

Mountain Rose Herbs, P.O. Box 2000, Redway, CA 95560. No charge for the mail-order catalog that lists herbs, books, oils, and bottles to package your own products and original medicinal tea blends.

Nature's Herb Company, 1010 46th Street, Emeryville, CA 94608. Now owned by Barry Meltzer since its esteemed former owner Nathan Podhurst passed away. The company has been moved to Emeryville from San Francisco. We all miss Nathan and Emma here in San Francisco but Emma is still at Nature's Herb Company and if you phone she will send you a free mail-order catalog. The parent company is San Francisco Herb & Natural Food. Retail and wholesale bulk herbs, teas, spices, essential oils, tinctures, extracts, etc.

Pacific Botanicals, 4350 Fish Hatchery Road, Grants Pass, OR 97527. Organically-grown herbs and spices sold both dried and fresh. No charge for price sheet. A fine company.

Phybiosis, P.O. Box 992, Bowie, MD 20718. This is a new source of top-quality essential oils at wholesale prices as well as wonderful healing clay distinguished by particular colors of green, red, yellow, pink, white. They also have a good quality diffusor and aromatherapy and herb products. Write for a catalog and tell them Jeanne Rose sent you.

Prima Fleur Botanicals, 1201 R Andersen Dr., San Rafael, CA 94901. A fine company for all your essential oils and especially freshly distilled hydrosols. They keep Rose-Geranium Lavender, Lavandin, Lemon-Verbena, and other hydrosols that are all therapeutically active. Phone (415) 455-0957.

Send a postcard to the sources listed here for more information. Call your *local women's health organization* to find out where to obtain a speculum.

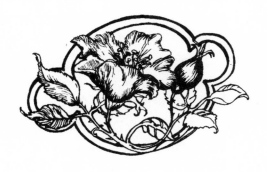

Bibliography

Beckett, Sarah. *Herbs for Feminine Ailments: Everybody's Home Herbal.* Wellingborough, Northamptonshire: Thorsons, 1973.
_____. *Herbs for Prostate and Bladder Troubles: Everybody's Home Herbal.* Wellingborough, Northamptonshire: Thorsons, 1973.

Donsbach, Kurt W., Ph.D., D.Sc., N.D., D.C. *Dr. Donsbach Tells You What You Always Wanted to Know About Menopause.* International Institute of Natural Health Sciences, Inc., 1979.

Federation of Feminist Women's Health Centers. *A New View of a Woman's Body: A Fully Illustrated Guide.* New York: Simon and Schuster, 1981.

Fredericks, Carlton, Ph.D. *Carlton Fredericks' Guide to Women's Nutrition: Dietary Advice for Women of All Ages.* New York: G. P. Putnam's Sons, 1988.

Gardner, Joy. *A Difficult Decision: A Compassionate Book About Abortion.* Ann Arbor, MI: McNaughton & Gunn, 1986.

Green, James. *The Male Herbal: Health Care for Men and Boys.* Freedom, CA: The Crossing Press, 1991.

Harding, M. Ester. *Women's Mysteries.* New York: Harper & Row, 1976.

Hoffman, David. *The Herbal Handbook: A User's Guide to Medical Herbalism*. Rochester, VT: Healing Arts Press, 1988.

Koehler, Nan. *Artemis Speaks: V.B.A.C. Stories and Natural Childbirth Information*. Occidental, CA: Jerald R. Brown, Inc, 1985.

Lett, AlexSandra. *Herbal Abortion*. No publisher listed. 1977.

Maberley, D. J. *The Plant Book*. Cambridge, NY: Cambridge University Press, 1989.

Mabey, Richard. *The New Age Herbalist*. New York: Macmillan Publishing Co., 1992.

Maddux, Hilary C. *Menstruation*. Philadelphia, PA: Banbury Books, Inc., 1981.

Price, Shirley. *Shirley Price's Aromatherapy Workbook*. Wellingborough, Northamptonshire: Thorsons, 1993.

Reuben, Carolyn, C. A., and Joan Priestley, M.D. *Essential Supplements for Women*. New York: Perigee Books, 1988.

Rose, Jeanne. *The Aromatherapy Book: Applications & Inhalations, Third Edition*. Berkeley, CA: North Atlantic Books, 1994.
_____. *Herbal Studies Course*, Chapter 23. San Francisco, CA: Herbal Studies Library, 1988.

Seaman, Barbara, and Gideon Seaman, M.D. *Women and the Crisis in Sex Hormones*. New York: Bantam Books, 1977.

Shapiro, Howard I., M.D. *The Birth Control Book: A Complete Guide for Men and Women*. New York: Avon Books, 1978.

Slick, Rosemary Gladstar. *Sage Healing Ways Series: Herbs for Menopause*. E. Barre, VT: SAGE, (n.d.).

Weiss, Kay, Editor. *Women's Health Care: A Guide to Alternatives.* Reston, VA: Reston Publishing Co., Inc., 1984.

Whitehouse, Capt. Geoffrey T. *Everywoman's Guide to Natural Health.* Wellingborough, Northamptonshire: Thorsons, 1974.

Periodicals

Mayer, Ruth. "12 Ways Not to Get Pregnant." *Mademoiselle* Magazine. (August 1993).

Sahley, Dr. Billie J. "Nutritional Support for Menopause." *Whole Foods.* (January 1989).

Steinman, David. "Treating Prostate Troubles." *Natural Health.* (November/December 1993).

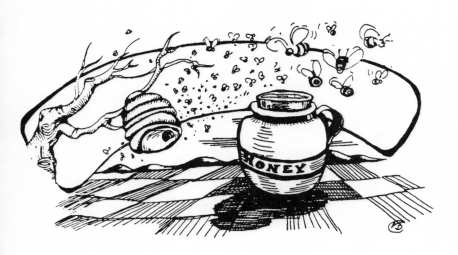

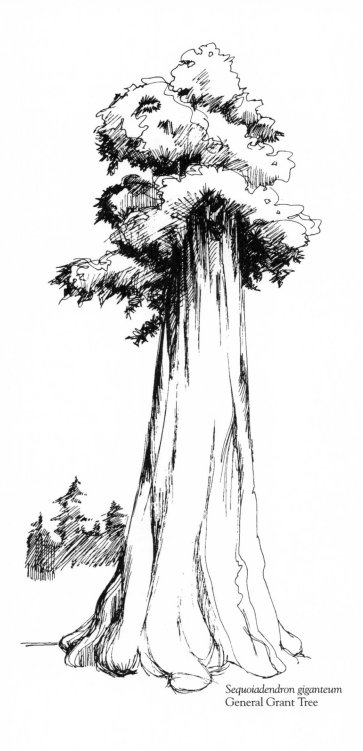

Sequoiadendron giganteum
General Grant Tree

About the Author

This California native daughter is an international authority on the therapeutic uses of herbs, both medicinal and cosmetic, and a well-known teacher of aromatherapy. The author of eight herbal books and an Herbal Studies Course by Correspondence, Ms. Rose has a rich familial and ethnic background in plant use. Jeanne's mother, Aline Lalancette, a beautiful French-Canadian woman, met Arsenio Colón through the lovelorn column of a New York newspaper in 1936. Ms. Lalancette boarded a transcontinental train just six weeks after their first letters were exchanged and married Mr. Colon in May 1936. Jeanne was born just eight months later. She grew up in the fertile valley of Contra Costa county on an Apricot orchard and from the first her days were filled with the natural experiences of country living and plant use. Jeanne graduated from the local schools, earned a degree in zoology at San Jose State College, and received a scholarship to the Marine Laboratory in Coral Gables, Florida. She worked in herbal and pesticide research at the Agricultural Experiment Stations in Florida, eventually relocating to her home state of California where she continued her private and public research into the medicinal uses of herbs and the therapeutic values of essential oils. Jeanne is an academic enthusiast and pursues her studies continually by personal and library research. She has a world-class personal library containing most of the important volumes in herbal studies and aromatherapy and is an inveterate reader.

Notes

Notes

Notes